The Student Nurse Handbook

Liz Aston and Lesley Strouther

 Open University Press

Open University Press
McGraw-Hill Education
McGraw-Hill House
Shoppenhangers Road
Maidenhead
Berkshire
England
SL6 2QL

email: enquiries@openup.co.uk
world wide web: www.openup.co.uk

and
Two Penn Plaza, New York, NY 10121-2289, USA

First published 2012

A catalogue record of this book is available from the British Library

ISBN13: 978-0-33-524475-1 (pb)
ISBN10: 0-33-524475-0 (pb)
eISBN: 978-0-33-524506-8

Library of Congress Cataloging-in-Publication Data
CIP data has been applied for

Typeset by Aptara Inc., India
Printed in the UK by Bell and Bain Ltd, Glasgow.

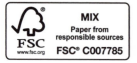

Contents

Introduction

This book is aimed at both individuals who are thinking about becoming a student nurse and students on a current programme. The idea for this book came from a group of nursing students at the University of Nottingham, who found there were lots of things they would have liked to have known about before starting their course. There were also lots of things at the beginning of their course that they hadn't expected.

We organized some focus groups with volunteer students so they could share what the main issues and concerns had been for them. From the information shared in these focus groups, we generated the chapters that form the basis of this book. Questions were then posted as an online survey that students from all fields of nursing and at different universities could complete. We received hundreds of responses representing what can be considered the valid views of existing students.

Chapter 1 addresses what nursing is from the students' perspective, Chapter 2 focuses on how to apply for the course of your choice and settling in, Chapters 3 and 4 explore getting the most out of your placement and the types of support available to you as a student. Placement issues are then dealt with in Chapter 5 followed by what it means to be an accountable practitioner in Chapter 6. Portfolios were highlighted in the focus groups as causing a lot of anxiety, so Chapter 7 includes lots of advice from students about how they have developed their portfolios. Chapter 8 addresses coming to the end of a course and how to apply for that first job.

It is important to remember that this book is driven by students' own experiences that they have willingly shared; it is the students' words you will read, written down with commentary by the authors.

We would like to thank all the students who have shared their experiences and thoughts and hope you enjoy reading their accounts.

1   What does it mean to be a nurse?

I became a healthcare assistant on the suggestion of my mother who is also a nurse, and immediately fell in love with nursing. It is my opinion that other professions such as physiotherapy or radiography do not provide the same opportunities to develop therapeutic relationships with patients as nursing does. There is a certain satisfaction gained from caring for people who are often unable to care for themselves and nursing allows me the privilege of caring for those people every day. (Child branch nursing student)

Topics covered in this chapter:

- Why people choose nursing as a career
- What caring means to nurses
- Choosing a particular branch of nursing
- How perceptions of what nursing is change
- Defining what nursing is
- What nursing means to students
- Finding out what to expect from a course
- Coping with a nursing programme
- Finding out about different nursing environments

Introduction

To be able to work in the health service in the UK, nurses must hold a degree or diploma in nursing (a 'pre-registration' programme), which will allow them to register with the Nursing and Midwifery Council (NMC), enabling them to practise as a nurse. Pre-registration degrees and diploma programmes are offered in four 'fields' of nursing: adult, child (paediatric), learning disability, and mental health. Most often, prospective students need to decide which of the four fields of nursing they wish to train for before making an application. A few higher education institutions may offer the flexibility of choosing a particular field of nursing after having started the course.

Why choose nursing as a career?

I chose nursing after experiencing the way that nurses can change lives and help to build people's confidence and help rebuild their lives.
(Mental health nursing student)

Previous work experience allowed me to view other professions and I felt that nursing was the one for me.
(Adult branch nursing student)

It [nursing] is more specific to patient care. I considered medicine but felt I would miss the interaction with patients and lose out on the opportunity to build professional relationships with them.
(Adult branch nursing student)

Because I enjoyed patient contact in my work experience and although I was offered places at med school, I felt there was little prolonged patient contact.
(Child branch nursing student)

Because I wanted to be able to look after those who were in mental distress, have that close contact that being a nurse enables but having a higher level of input than a healthcare assistant.
(Mental health nursing student)

Because I am a caring person who wants to be able to treat both physical problems and mental health problems within my profession.
(Mental health nursing student)

People often find it difficult to articulate why they choose nursing as a career but key to the above students' insights are that they want to be a nurse, want prolonged contact with people, want variety in their career, and identify that caring is central to being a nurse.

What does caring mean?

Caring in relation to nursing does not just mean providing physical care in the sense of washing and feeding. Nurses should genuinely have an interest in the health and wellbeing of their patients and want them to achieve good health, not just go through the motions of restoring physical health. If you don't care about helping those that need it, then you're in the wrong profession.

(Adult branch nursing student)

Caring is vital in the nursing profession. It's what drives a nurse to give good care and make people better. It makes clients feel valued and that they've had a positive experience. Caring means having people's best concerns at heart and demonstrating this by your actions for and towards the person.

(Mental health nursing student)

I think caring almost defines nursing and can be shown in many ways, from providing basic hygiene care to listening to a family member or advocating for someone when necessary.

(Child branch nursing student)

Caring means considering all aspects of the situation. The patient's wishes, religious beliefs, what is best for the patient, the support needed, supporting the family, providing adequate and understandable information. You must be sympathetic and understanding yet remain professional.

(Child branch nursing student)

Caring means doing the best for your patient. It involves building a relationship with the patient by showing empathy, compassion, and sensitivity. It involves taking a genuine interest in the patient to make them feel important and respected.

(Adult branch nursing student)

'Caring' encompasses a multitude of things and actions – talking to patients, understanding their preferences, protecting and promoting their personal dignity, supporting their choices, individualizing your approach to best suit your patient ... I could go on, as the list would be ever-changing and endless!

(Adult branch nursing student)

Caring means showing empathy, patience, listening, and respecting people. It means always doing your best for the person and sometimes it means allowing that person to make mistakes and support them on their road to recovery. Sometimes those who care the most are the ones that step back and allow patients to make their own choices – whether we agree or not – and be the ones who support them and encourage them to try again if they fail the first time.

(Mental health nursing student)

Caring to me is not only providing an individual with the assistance he or she needs to survive, but to also promote independence, maintain psychological well-being, whilst being a figure of trust, support, and security to all patients.

(Adult branch nursing student)

Caring is being dependable, trustworthy, and understanding what an individual wants and needs and helping them to obtain it or achieve it.
(Learning disability nursing student)

Caring is an essential component of nursing with nursing being a complex and unique relationship between patient and nurse (Sumner 2001). It involves feeling on the part of the nurse, which can make the nurse feel vulnerable just as a patient can feel vulnerable (Henderson 2001). Nurses can become emotionally engaged with patients and need to know how to balance caring and involvement with being a professional nurse. This is what you need to learn throughout your nursing programme, observing the nurses you work with to help you to interpret for yourself what makes a caring, compassionate but professional nurse. McCormack and McCance (2006) identify four important aspects in delivering care to people, the first of which is the personal attributes of the nurse. McCormack and McCance (2006) also highlight that in order to care you need to be committed to the nursing role, have good interpersonal skills, be empathetic, have good social skills, and have an awareness of yourself as a person.

ACTIVITY 1.1

Think about your own personal attributes.

- Do you possess these personal attributes?
- How can you work on/develop these?
- How will awareness of yourself help you to decide which branch of nursing to choose?

Why choose a particular field of nursing?

I researched the different branches to find the one which I felt suited my personality and career goals.

(Adult branch nursing student)

I have always enjoyed working with children and also working in the community. Children's nursing seemed a good way to combine those.
(Child branch nursing student)

I thought it would be to hard to see children ill and even worse dying, so I opted for adult nursing. However, after experiencing nursing I have learnt that it doesn't matter what age or their circumstances – it's still hard to see.
(Adult branch nursing student)

I have worked with children and adults with learning disabilities and mental health problems in other settings within healthcare and would like to work with a variety of different people now. I imagined that if I chose the adult branch I would work with the whole mix of people, which so far has been true.
(Adult branch nursing student)

I have been working in learning disabilities for the last few years, and want to make a difference for the people I have met along the way.
(Learning disabilities nursing student)

I visited a range of open days and researched the areas I could work in within each branch. Although very interested in child nursing, I opted for adult as I felt my skills best met the requirements of an adult nurse and felt excited by the range of areas I could work in once qualified.
(Adult branch nursing student)

I've got people in my family who suffer from mental health issues … Also, I find there is a stigma against people who suffer from mental health problems, which I don't agree with and I want to be one of the nurses who tries to break the stigma.
(Mental health nursing student)

I have always been interested in people. I watched how a nurse helped a teenager I knew, over the course of a few months and wanted to be able to make that sort of a difference to people's lives.
(Mental health nursing student)

Through babysitting for many different aged children, volunteering in primary and secondary schools I knew I wanted a career working with children. A great sense of achievement can be gained through helping someone and providing support to overcome something. Personally I feel I can gain much more from working with a family unit which is what children's nursing involves.
(Child branch nursing student)

Key elements that the above students identify include:

- researching the different fields of nursing;
- having previous experience of healthcare;
- variety of work;
- personal experiences.

   Researching which field is right for you is really important. You need to find out what nurses in each field do to make sure it is what you want to do. For example, some individuals think that the child field involves simply looking after children and babies but as one student explained, it is about looking after the family unit, not just the child. However, your own personal experiences or prior experience in healthcare settings can also help you to identify what is right for you. All fields of nursing offer an incredible variety of experiences and opportunities, and the Nursing and Midwifery Council (NMC 2010) recognize that most skills that nurses need to acquire are the same for each of the four fields. Hall and Ritchie (2009) asked qualified nurses what each field of nursing is about, see Chapter 7 of their book for more information.

How do students' perceptions of what nursing is change with experience?

Before finding out what mental health nursing involved specifically I was quite ignorant to the job role. The stereotype of a nurse working on a medical ward was what I envisioned when I heard the term.
                                                    (Mental health nursing student)

I realized that the focus of nursing between the branches is very different. Clearly in mental health nursing, nursing skills in the form of addressing physical health problems are still vital and utilized in practice, but the focus was on forming therapeutic relationships with people and spending time with them rather than the job being so task-orientated.
                                                    (Mental health nursing student)

Helping adults in diverse settings to improve/safeguard their health. It's a lot tougher emotionally than I realized. There is greater diversity of roles than I imagined, even within the same care setting. I had been prepared for it to be hard, unglamorous, physical work, and it is!
                                                    (Adult branch nursing student)

I thought nursing was about caring for patients with varied health backgrounds in either acute care or critical. I thought nursing was about administering medications, and liaising with doctors on further care they may need. My perception changed a lot. I didn't realize the amount of paperwork a nurse had to do, how much was documented and the amount of responsibility the nurse actually has.

(Adult branch nursing student)

I never imagined just how hard nurses have to work. Twelve and a half hour shifts and they are on their feet for almost twelve of those hours on some of the wards I've worked on. It is very tiring.

(Adult branch nursing student)

Supporting individuals to lead positive lives. That it is going to be a tougher job then I expected to make a difference.

(Learning disability nursing student)

I didn't really realize how many different things nurses had to organize, i.e. social sort outs and referrals. I didn't realize how many members of the MDT [multidisciplinary team] there are. Naively, I truly believed it was about just caring for sick patients.

(Adult branch nursing student)

I realized there was more than just caring for a poorly patient – it was how everything I did had an impact on them, their families, carers, friends, other nursing staff but, most importantly, I never realized how important it was as a nurse to care for yourself while caring for others both mentally and physically.

(Mental health nursing student)

I realized the full range of skills required to be an adult nurse and the fact that the nurse cares for the patient, their family and their loved ones, not just the patient. Additionally, I learnt quickly that the nurse is an advocate for the patient and is required to understand a real breadth of theory to enable them to provide evidence-based care.

(Adult branch nursing student)

Talking through people's problems, giving them medication, taking them out and helping them to learn skills to cope. My perception did change because I felt I went into nursing thinking it was a lot easier than it was – I didn't realize how clever you had to be and how many skills you needed to deliver effective patient care.

(Mental health nursing student)

I realized I would be dealing with a variety of illnesses but also that, with an ageing population, there would be a lot of elderly care and the illnesses and conditions specific to an older age group.

(Adult branch nursing student)

Caring for not only children aged 0–19 but also for their parents and siblings. Although daunting at first, my placements have been very rewarding. While carrying out routine observations on an 8-year-old boy he asked me to explain how I could feel his heart beat, so while counting his radial pulse I explained to him that I was feeling the strength of his heart and counting how many times it was beating. I then showed him how to feel it – his face lit up when he did. He then went on to try and find his mum's pulse. This small experience made my day as I felt that not only had I gained but he also had learnt something and was smiling and happy even though he was in hospital.

(Child branch nursing student)

Providing nursing care for adults of all ages, I knew this would some-times include patients with either mental health conditions or learn-ing disabilities with either surgical or medical admissions. I thought of nursing as providing basic care, as well as giving out medications and working with doctors and other healthcare professionals to meet spe-cific goals for each patient. Most of it was what I had expected, but I was surprised how different two wards could be. I realized that even for qualified nurses they are still continuously learning new skills and methods of providing care.

(Adult branch nursing student)

It's not as glamorous as television programmes make out!

(Adult branch nursing student)

I thought that the majority of children I worked with would be critically ill but during the course you get to work in respite homes, medical wards, surgical wards and out in the community. The types of children you come into contact with varies between placements; they could be disabled, have learning difficulties, mental/psychological problems, long-term medical conditions, self-inflicted injuries – the list goes on.

(Child branch nursing student)

It is clear from the above comments that, while the main focus of each of the fields may differ, all fields of nursing involve physical, psychological, social, and emotional support and care for both the patient/service user and the significant people in their lives. Nursing involves a lot of hard work and is not the glamorous profession that is portrayed in the media at times. When caring for patients it can be emotionally and physically draining and you need to care for yourself. To do this you need to have good support mechanisms both within and outside the profession, en-suring you look after yourself both physically and emotionally. However, nursing can be an extremely rewarding profession that involves:

- responsibility;
- the importance of documenting care;
- being a team worker alongside other members of the healthcare team;
- the need to acquire theoretical knowledge in order to deliver effective nursing care;
- the need for health promotion skills to enable people to make informed choices in their lives;
- the need for lifelong learning about nursing to ensure your care delivery is up to date.

These are all key elements that help to identify and define what it means to be a nurse.

Defining what nursing is

Nursing is aimed at making the lives of people who are in need better. It is about helping people while they are ill, helping them throughout recovery, and helping them maintain their health. It's about assisting people achieve better health and a better quality of life through using their knowledge, skills, and compassion.

(Mental health nursing student)

Nursing to me is a way to help others, not only heal people both inside and out but an opportunity to use one of life's greatest skills – communication – to help put a smile on someone's face, to helping them deal with terminal illness and great losses.

(Adult branch nursing student)

Nursing is not a glamorous job but hardworking and [you] need to be dedicated in providing the best possible care. At times you are surrounded by challenges, lack of time, and lack of recourses. An attempt to help heal the ill and wounded in diverse situations everywhere you go. Stepping in to people's lives and offer support advice and educate when needed.

(Adult branch nursing student)

Caring for people of all types in an educated, non-prejudicial, and informed way to provide the best outcomes for them. Not just in hospital but in numerous places within communities.

(Learning disability nursing student)

Nursing has never been just a job, it is no longer a vocation; it is, however, a profession. A profession that requires commitment beyond that of any other, and one which provides the greatest of rewards.
(Learning disability nursing student)

Nursing is about being there for your patients. It is about working professionally and using the best evidence-based research to care for each patient. It is about seeing each patient as an individual and tailoring care to suit their needs. It is about providing the BEST care possible.
(Mental health nursing student)

It is a holistic approach to medicine involving the care of the physical and psychological wellbeing of patients.
(Adult branch nursing student)

Caring for a person who is in need, looking at them holistically. Caring can be to look after someone with the goal of making them better, or it could be through to death to try and make it a comfortable and peaceful one.
(Adult branch nursing student)

Nursing, in paediatrics, is the care of a child and his or her family, whoever that may be – mum, dad, grandmother, uncle, teddy, family friend, and wherever that care may be required – hospital, school, at home, in the park, so that the child and his or her family may thrive to his/her full potential.
(Child branch nursing student)

Nursing is not just about dishing out tablets and helping people wash. Yes, it is helping people to help themselves get better and caring for those who can't care for themselves, but it is also being there for your patients in any way you can when they need you.
(Adult branch nursing student)

To be part of the nursing profession requires a caring, compassionate approach in which the care delivered needs to meet all patients' needs as well as the needs of their family members/significant others. The above students refer to helping patients towards recovery or through to a peaceful and dignified death. There are more official definitions of nursing. The International Council of Nurses (2011) define nursing as follows:

Nursing encompasses autonomous and collaborative care of individuals of all ages, families, groups and communities, sick or well and in all settings. Nursing includes the promotion of health, prevention of illness, and the care of ill, disabled and dying people. Advocacy, promotion of a safe environment, research, participation in shaping health policy and in patient and health systems management, and education are also key nursing roles.

The students' comments within this chapter reflect this definition of nursing well. Within the UK, the Royal College of Nursing (RCN 2011) define nursing as:

> the use of clinical judgement in the provision of care to enable people to improve, maintain, or recover health, to cope with health problems, and to achieve the best possible quality of life, whatever the disease or disability, until death.

These definitions of nursing bring together a lot of the students' observations about what nursing is and highlight the underpinning principles of what it means to be a nurse. Nursing is a challenging undertaking requiring full commitment on the part of individuals who want to be part of the profession.

What does being a nurse mean?

It means striving to do the best by and for the patient, trying to act as if it were my family member in the bed daily. I was unprepared for the sense of responsibility and the amount of trust placed in you by both the patient and their family.
(Adult branch nursing student)

It means being a professional with an important role to play within healthcare. It means being accountable for my practice. It means providing the best available care for my patients.
(Adult branch nursing student)

Everything, it is so pleasurable to me knowing I have made a positive impact on somebody else's lifestyle. I feel I give myself respect and trust at the same time when helping or caring for somebody.
(Mental health nursing student)

It means having an opportunity to support people in a way that really makes a difference to their lives. It makes me feel that I am very fortunate and privileged to be a part of people's lives for a while during the most difficult and tragic times they will go through.
(Child branch nursing student)

It means helping people to move on. To maybe not become someone different, but accept all of their mental health issues and learn to live

*with them in a way that is functional and appropriate to them. Giving
something back and helping.*

(Mental health nursing student)

Key points the above students highlight include:

- helping people;
- being trustworthy;
- taking responsibility;
- being accountable for your actions.

As a nurse, you need to be honest and trustworthy. The people you
nurse are often vulnerable individuals who are dependent on you to act
in a caring, compassionate, and professional manner. As a nurse, you also
have to take responsibility for providing effective nursing care for your
client group and the profession provides a lot of guidance for nurses in
how to behave and what their responsibilities are (see further reading list
at the end of the chapter).

During your nursing programme, you will be supervised and during
this time you need to learn as much as you can from the staff you work
with in practice. In addition, you need to have a good knowledge and
skills base that will help you learn to make the right decisions about
patient care as well being able to deliver that care safely. This is why the
practice element of the course is so important. As a nurse, you also have
to be accountable for the care you deliver, which means being able to
explain why you chose a specific action and what evidence base you used
to decide on that particular action in a given situation. This is something
you will learn to do during your nursing course with the help of your
lecturing staff and practitioners you work alongside.

Finding out what to expect from a course

*I found out through a friend that was planning on entering the profes-
sion. I also found out by researching the job role of a mental health
nurse. I also looked at the university's course prospectus.*

(Mental health nursing student)

*Open days and my interview – but I don't feel like I knew what to expect
until I started the course.*

(Child branch nursing student)

*I undertook an access to higher education course at my local college,
which helped to prepare me for the course.*

(Adult branch nursing student)

Speaking to others within the healthcare settings; however, I don't think anyone can really prepare you for how demanding this course can be on your life for the three years it takes.

(Adult branch nursing student)

The university website, talking to people who had recently done the course or who were already doing it.

(Learning disability nursing student)

Online at NHS.uk and at the university website.

(Adult branch nursing student)

I attended open days, which provided me with the opportunity to speak to current students, past students, current health professionals, and lecturers. I looked on the student room forum to see comments from other students as well to gain a larger picture.

(Child branch nursing student)

It is obviously useful to find out about what to expect from a course. Nursing programmes are not like other university courses. At the end of your programme, you will have both an academic degree as well as a vocational qualification. This means the course is extremely demanding and, as the students identify, it is difficult to prepare yourself for how demanding it can be. Make sure you find out as much as you can before you commit yourself, as undertaking a nursing programme, although extremely rewarding, is a real challenge. Most university courses are solely academic programmes, requiring attendance at university for lectures with the rest of the time available for studying and other activities. A nursing programme requires you to spend time in practice learning to look after patients/service users, as well as time in university learning to be effective in practice. In addition, nursing students must have competed 2300 hours in practice and 2300 hours in academic study. The academic element will involve attending university for classes as well as self-directed study. The practice element, on the other hand, will involve practice experience in diverse clinical settings that expose you to all parts of the patient's journey through the health and social care system.

Coping with a nursing programme

It's a very steep learning curve, especially while trying to be a student nurse, get the work done, earn some money, and have as good and as normal a 'student life' as possible. It probably didn't hit me until I got my first mediocre result and then I realized, but you just have to be able to discipline yourself and learn what you can cope with and work within those limits.

(Child branch nursing student)

With difficulty. Dedicating time to university work is important, but setting aside time to relax and forget about it is even more so. It can take over your life if you're not careful.

(Adult branch nursing student)

It can be tough juggling all the requirements that this course throws at you as well as managing life away from Uni. As a mature student, I have a mortgage and bills to pay, which requires some very careful financial planning!

(Adult branch nursing student)

To be honest, I think just about cope is accurate!! I am a mum of three, so balancing home work and study is vital. I don't do any housework that isn't very necessary until the holidays. I make use of any spare moment at work to write up or research for the outcomes. I make sure the children get time with me each day and I study every weekday even if only for half an hour, just to keep a routine!

(Mental health nursing student)

Take advantage of all the support networks that are made available . . . from a chat with my mum to a deep discussion with a tutor.

(Adult branch nursing student)

I found it very difficult to begin with. This was mainly due to having an unidentified learning need throughout the first year. Since having this diagnosed, I have accessed student support and received the appropriate help. I now have very good coping strategies for completing assignment work.

(Adult branch nursing student)

Organizing, making sure I know when things need to be done by, asking the people around me to support me, letting them know what I need to achieve my goals and how they can support that.

(Learning disability nursing student)

I'm still getting to the grips of adjusting in some ways and I don't think I ever will fully adjust. It's an extremely testing course, but worthwhile in the long run. I tend to focus on my goal of achieving and somehow get through that way.

(Mental health nursing student)

I think I have learned to cope with the help of other students. We are quite close as a group and there is always someone to help, by letting me moan or by giving me a kick up the backside when it is needed.

(Adult branch nursing student)

I didn't. I had a wealth of experience working with children, but I was so busy with A levels and then 'volunteering' up to a week before my course started I didn't give myself enough time to prepare for what the course might be like. Fortunately, I loved it, but I can see why so many people drop out.

(Child branch nursing student)

I think it definitely helped to have some healthcare experience before the course, as the shift patterns can be a big shock to those who've never worked in healthcare. Also, the more basic tasks such as washing a patient and being with them in their final hours can be daunting to people fresh into healthcare.

(Adult branch nursing student)

I had no experience whatsoever in the field of nursing or healthcare. I was a civil servant for 15 years and then a stay-at-home mum. I went into nursing with very little knowledge. I feel that maybe some healthcare work prior to staring the course may have helped, but I'm doing just fine without it, so it's not essential.

(Adult branch nursing student)

Yes, I knew more what to expect at the basic level of care provision, understood some of the terms used, understood it wasn't going to be a walk in the park, that there would be a lot of work and that it would be physically and mentally challenging.

(Learning disability nursing student)

I had personal experience of being with a mental health nurse in the community, however I wasn't prepared for it at all. It came as a shock to the system, but the support you receive is enough to settle you in and calm you down if you're anxious!

(Mental health nursing student)

From the above quotes it is clear that prior experience can help in some ways. However, as other students point out who didn't have previous experience, they coped well with the demands of the course. The main things to bear in mind are what nurses have to do on a daily basis and the fact that you will need to find time to study and write academic assignments, as well as the need to have a social life.

Key points to think about include:

- the need for self-discipline in terms of balancing your personal life with academic and practice demands;
- time management is essential – deadlines for assignments mean you need to plan and organize your time, not leave things until the last minute;
- support – take whatever support is offered. Support systems need to include your family, friends, other students, and the lecturing staff. Don't be too proud to ask for help or leave asking for help until you reach crisis point.

Earning some money to supplement the financial help available while on the course is an option most students have to take. However, you need to balance additional work with meeting the demands of the course and this is something that all students need to think about before starting a nursing programme. In addition, some universities provide guidance about how much paid work students should undertake outside their programme of study. As will be clear from the students' comments above, this can be especially difficult for those with dependents, who will experience extra demands on their time and finances, such as for child care.

Finding out about different nursing environments

I was always aware of health visitors and school nurses just through my experiences in younger life, but I had never considered that placements like these would make up such a huge proportion of my practice placements.

(Child branch nursing student)

During the course and from speaking to other students after their different placements.

(Adult branch nursing student)

Internet and friends.

(Mental health nursing student)

Health and social care 'A level' covered the different roles and health settings of a nurse.

(Child branch nursing student)

I found that the biggest difference was that I was used to being independent when working, and when I went on placement I was supervised at all times doing things that I had been competent at for some time.

(Adult branch nursing student)

By working in them! You have no idea how wide the scope of nursing is until you start being sent to placement areas you hadn't even considered.
(Child branch nursing student)

I already had a good understanding of the services out there, but the course website, open days, and reading were all helpful.
(Learning disabilities nursing student)

The settings in which nurses are required to deliver care are diverse. Settings include:

- inpatient care (e.g. in a hospital);
- community care (e.g. in a patient's own home, a GP surgery or day centres);
- charitable services (e.g. hospices or working with the homeless);
- private care services (e.g. nursing homes, private hospitals or private community services);
- social care settings (e.g. residential care).

Nursing offers many opportunities to you. If you are considering nursing or are already on a nursing course, make the most of all the learning opportunities on offer. As part of your programme you need to have experience of, and insight into, the pathway through the healthcare system that the patient experiences. You will have placements in diverse health and social care settings that will enable you to explore the role of a nurse in a particular setting. Your practice experiences will also provide you with an understanding of how different health and social care workers contribute to effective care for patients, and how important it is for all professions to work collaboratively for the benefit of patients using the health service.

Key points covered in this chapter

- Students' perspectives on why they chose nursing as a career
- Students' views on what caring means to a nurse
- Things to consider about which field of nursing to choose
- Students' perspectives on what nursing means for them
- Definitions of what nursing is
- Things to expect from a nursing course

References

Hall, C. and Ritchie, D. (2009) *What is Nursing? Exploring Theory and Practice*. Exeter: Learning Matters.

Henderson, A. (2001) Emotional labor and nursing: an under-appreciated aspect of caring work, *Nursing Inquiry*, 8(2): 130–8.

International Council of Nurses (2011) http://www.icn.ch/about-icn/icn-definition-of-nursing (accessed 21 April 2011).

McCormack, B. and McCance, T.V. (2006) Development of a framework for person-centred nursing, *Journal of Advanced Nursing*, 56(5): 472–9.

Nursing and Midwifery Council (NMC) (2010) *Standards for Pre-registration Nursing Education*. London: NMC. Available at: http://standards.nmc-uk.org/PublishedDocuments/Standards%20for%20pre-registration%20nursing%20education%2016082010.pdf

Royal College of Nursing (RCN) (2011) rcn-uk.org (accessed 21 April 2011).

Sumner, J. (2001) Caring in nursing: a different interpretation, *Journal of Advanced Nursing*, 35(6): 926–32.

Further reading

Nursing and Midwifery Council (NMC) (2008) *The Code: Standards of Conduct, Performance and Ethics for Nurses and Midwives*. London: NMC.

Nursing and Midwifery Council (NMC) (2010a) *Good Health and Good Character: Guidance for Approved Education Institutions*. London: NMC.

Nursing and Midwifery Council (NMC) (2010b) *Raising and Escalating Concerns: Guidance for Nurses and Midwives*. London: NMC.

2 Preparing to undertake the course

> *Nursing requires a great deal more stamina and dedication than other university courses. Not only do you have to balance the theory with the practical but you also have to make sure you maintain your attendance in both, something that's not required for graduation from other courses.*
> (Adult branch nursing student)

Topics covered in this chapter:

- Preparing to study
- How to choose a place to study
- What open days can offer
- How to apply for nursing through UCAS
- Writing a personal statement
- Applying for funding
- Settling in during the early days of the course
- What self-directed learning means
- How to balance nursing with home and social life

Introduction

The main focus of this chapter is on preparing you for your application to university to study to become a registered nurse. Existing students share their experiences of pre-nursing study, applying for the course, and obtaining funding. Once accepted into their chosen field of nursing, student nurses provide insight into their early days of the course and approaches to learning. Finally, the chapter offers a brief insight into how the new student nurse balances studying with a home and social life.

Meeting pre-registration nursing study requirements

The requirement at the time I applied for nursing was five GCSEs grade C and above. I did, however, find having work experience through completing my BTEC National Qualification helped me secure my place.

(Adult branch nursing student)

I had already completed a degree and I was clear about the academic study expected from a university course in nursing.

(Adult branch nursing student)

I did a one-year access course prior to starting my degree. I needed to top up my grades but I also felt that as I had not been in education for some time, it would give me a chance to 'break myself in' a bit and see if I could cope with the demands of the degree course.

(Child branch nursing student)

I did NVQ Level II in Health and Social Care and I also obtained my maths and English skills through learndirect.

(Adult branch nursing student)

Universities in England, Scotland, Wales, and Northern Ireland advertise their pre-registration courses on the Internet and produce informative brochures for potential applicants. Individual universities can determine the minimum level of qualifications required by applicants but this must be based on the guidance issued by the Nursing and Midwifery Council (NMC). The NMC is the professional regulatory body for nurses and midwives and its principal aim is to protect and safeguard the general public. In setting standards for education, the NMC seeks to ensure nursing and midwifery students have the right skills and qualities before they start work (NMC 2008). The latest 'Standards for Pre-registration Nursing Education' document was published in 2010 and replaces the 2004 guidance for the Diploma in nursing course. Visit the NMC website for the most up-to-date information on the minimum entry requirements.

Some students enter pre-registration nursing with the more traditional forms of school qualifications, such as GCSEs and A levels, but other educational equivalents may be considered. Many colleges of further education have recognized full- and part-time study programmes. The BTEC Level 2 Diploma in Health and Social Care, for example, is regulated by EDEXCEL and is broadly equivalent to four GCSEs grades A–C (BTEC 2011). In contrast, learndirect provides an online study programme in numeracy and/or literacy to certificate level within three months, which allows prospective students to top up GCSE grades to the required minimum standard for entry (learndirect 2011).

Many universities also ask for evidence of recent study, and nursing – unlike some other university programmes – appeals to individuals of all ages. The 'access course' mentioned by one of the students above is more formally named the Access to Higher Education and Nursing course, and is designed for adults who have been out of education for some time and want to demonstrate recent learning and enrol on a university level course (NHS Careers 2011). It is worth considering whether such a course or something similar could help you to be a successful applicant.

Choosing a place to study

Choosing the university in which to study nursing is a key decision. An undergraduate pre-registration course is typically three years in duration and for some the choice of where to study will be simply one of practicality. If you are a mature student or have a partner and/or children, you may consider your options limited to one of the nearest and therefore most convenient places to study. Others will not be so restricted and will be able to explore more fully their choices before deciding to apply. The NMC offers a directory of places to study nursing, which you can access via their website (http://www.nmc-uk.org/Approved-Programmes/). You can explore the potential higher education providers, request learning prospectuses, and find out about any open days.

What open days can offer

An open day 'is when members of the public may visit a place or institution to which they do not usually have access' (*The Oxford Dictionary* 2011).

> *I had no qualms about deciding on the right course and attending open days helped me decide on the right university. You have to make sure that you pick the right university; even if you don't move away from home, university becomes your second home, so you need to make sure you feel comfortable spending lots of time there.*
> (Adult branch nursing student)

> *On my open day I got a feel for the environment and gained information I needed to make an informed choice about the course I wanted to do.*
> (Mental health nursing student)

I attended several open days at different universities and found them really helpful. Open days provide you with the opportunity to take a look around the university, meet lecturers, talk to current staff, and generally get the feel of the course.

(Child branch nursing student)

I attended many open days in order to decide which university I wanted to attend. I visited the university I chose three times prior to accepting my place to learn more about the facilities and accommodation. At the open day I spoke to current students who gave a true representation of the course. By speaking to existing students, you will get a more accurate picture of the course and essentially how your life will change.

(Child branch nursing student)

I decided not to attend an open day. The course and the information on the website made available by the university was sufficient.

(Adult branch nursing student)

Open days allow a university to demonstrate the strengths of the pre-nursing course they are offering. Often, several open days are provided over a calendar year. In addition to receiving written information and pamphlets, attending an open day provides the prospective candidate with an opportunity to visit the university's School of Nursing and, if appropriate, the halls of residence with their parents or partner. An open day is an excellent opportunity for you to question lecturing staff and existing students about the university, the course, and the potential for post-registration employment. Once you start the application process, you will be asked to indicate the field of nursing you are interested in, thus attending open days and talking to lecturers and students will help you in making this decision.

Many universities conduct interviews to select candidates for nursing, so attending an open day is a good way of preparing yourself for questions that may be asked at interview, such as:

- What do you understand about the course you are applying for?
- Why choose nursing?
- Why have you chosen the specific field of nursing?
- What does nursing mean to you?

Applying for nursing through UCAS

I telephoned the university I wished to study at to ask if they had places on the course before I applied and they told me to apply through UCAS.

(Adult branch nursing student)

I was studying for a Health and Social Care diploma at college, so naturally we had talks about applying to university through UCAS.
(Adult branch nursing student)

I found out about applying through UCAS by accessing the course information in the university prospectus.
(Adult branch nursing student)

I was advised by the careers advisor to apply via UCAS.
(Mental health nursing student)

Almost all full-time education programmes at universities and colleges use the clearing system, the Universities and Colleges Admissions Service (UCAS). Many potential students are aware of the application process but, as is evident, some prospective students seek guidance from teachers, career advisors such as Connexions, or through contacting the pre-registration course provider directly. Connexions is now part of Directgov: Young People and offers free advice and access to a local Connexions advisor for anyone aged 13–19 years (Department for Education 2011).

UCAS is a standardized online approach to applying for a place on a course at university (UCAS 2011b). The application process is relatively simple but there is a telephone number for you to use should you need guidance. It may not be possible to apply when you feel ready; there are certain times at which courses are made available and there is a charge made for applying to a university. Career advisors, further education teachers, and admissions staff at a specific university will be able to advise you when to apply for your pre-registration nursing course. There is, however, an opportunity to apply for a nursing course at more than one university and for more than one field of nursing through UCAS.

I had some help through the booklets given to me by my college, which explained the process of applying and what to put in your personal statement. Information like that is extremely useful.
(Adult branch nursing student)

Help was available but I found the process relatively simple so I didn't require the extensive support.
(Child branch nursing student)

I rang [UCAS] once with a query and they talked me through what I needed to do.
(Adult branch nursing student)

Writing a personal statement

College provided us with help. They read over our personal statements, but they didn't help with the actual data side of the application, for example checking UCAS codes for different universities and courses.
(Child branch nursing student)

We had practice at writing our personal statements in college, which was good but didn't set the same restrictions as the UCAS form does – that is, word count – so I ended up submitting something quite different.
(Child branch nursing student)

I received help at sixth-form college from my tutor. However, through accessing the UCAS website I was able to find out more information. I also pulled up the university prospectus to help me write my personal statement. Ask friends and family who have done it before; even if they haven't, ask them to check your spelling!
(Child branch nursing student)

Universities shortlist suitable applicants for pre-registration nursing courses and then either offer them a place directly or an interview. Students preparing to apply may ask for guidance from teachers, friends and family members, and elsewhere. A university course prospectus will provide indicators of what the entry profile is and suggestions for the content of your personal statement. There is general guidance on the UCAS website regarding personal statements, where they state (UCAS 2011a):

Some course tutors find personal statements crucial when making decisions, whereas others might not put as much emphasis on them. Since you do not know who will be looking at your statement, the safest thing is to do a good job.

ACTIVITY 2.1

Writing your personal statement

- Obtain a university prospectus and read the guidelines on writing a personal statement.
- Look at your strengths and match these to the qualities in the prospectus.
- Consider what nursing is and means to you (see Chapter 1).
- Reflect on your previous experience and how you can use the skills and qualities you have developed when providing nursing care.

- Do you have any previous care experiences that you can include in your statement?
- How can you demonstrate caring and compassion?
- Can you demonstrate that you understand the demands of a pre-registration nursing course?
- Is there anything else that you could include, such as undertaking voluntary work at home or abroad?

Applying for financial help

I was made aware at the open day that course fees were paid and I was entitled to a student bursary. I was told the form to apply for this would be sent out with confirmation of receiving a place.

(Child branch nursing student)

I found out about tuition fees and bursary through the university web pages, prospectus and, finally, when I was offered a place.

(Adult branch nursing student)

I found out about accessing financial support by accessing the NHS website.

(Adult branch nursing student)

And once we started the course, we were informed by the student union what other funding is available.

(Adult branch nursing student)

Financial support is important to all students. Student nurses undertaking a Diploma in Nursing currently have their student fees paid by the NHS Business Services Authority (NHSBSA) and receive a bursary starting at £6701 per annum as per the *NHS Bursary Scheme, Twelfth Edition* (Department of Health 2011). The NHS Business Services Authority administers bursaries for healthcare students on behalf of the Department of Health (NHSBSA 2011). The information, terms, and conditions for student bursaries are updated each year. It is important that you read the terms and conditions before applying for the bursary payment.

The first day of the course

I was so nervous! I hardly slept the night before and it was terrifying arriving on day one . . . but after I arrived, I quickly made friends and settled in.

(Adult branch nursing student)

Felt like a dream until I got my badge with 'student nurse' on it, then it sunk in.

(Child branch nursing student)

Felt scared – but at least everyone else was in the same boat.

(Child branch nursing student)

The first day is a blur ... The strongest memory I have is being shocked at how many of us were there and the overwhelming sense of tiredness – and this was just theory, not even placement yet.

(Adult branch nursing student)

I was excited to be starting but felt overwhelmed and daunted by the size of both the cohort and the university.

(Adult branch nursing student)

Student nurse places are commissioned and universities are advised of how many students they are required to train to meet the demand for newly registered nurses. There are four fields of nursing: adult, child (paediatric), mental health, and learning disabilities. The first few days or weeks of a course allow for the induction and orientation processes, sometimes know as 'freshers'. The purpose of freshers is to help you familiarize yourself with university life and your surroundings. Starting a new course brings a mixture of emotions, such as excitement and apprehension. This has been recognized by the learning institutions, which have put in place wide-ranging support systems.

Introducing student support

The student union representative came to speak to us on the first day and provided us with small cards that had contact numbers and email addresses if we needed support.

(Child branch nursing student)

The university offers support – student support, counselling services, etc. – I didn't need to access them but it's reassuring knowing that I could if I need to.

(Adult branch nursing student)

You were allocated a personal tutor who would be with you all through university if ever you needed any help or advice.

(Adult branch nursing student)

My personal tutor was very good . . . The other teachers were good too, they had a lot of time for you to listen and explain and you never felt like you were bothering them.

(Mental health nursing student)

I had support from my peers. I feel the personal tutor system is poor. Some of my colleagues have personal tutors who take a great interest in them and see them on a regular basis, but I consider seeing your tutor twice a year is not conducive to a therapeutic relationship.

(Adult branch nursing student)

I was offered support by a student, a second-year buddy.

(Child branch nursing student)

The personal tutor fulfils key academic and pastoral functions. He or she provides a clear point of contact and is therefore seen by many students as pivotal to their progress and development. Registered nurses are encouraged to think holistically about their learning and progress and can create an integrated support system for themselves and others. Encouraging student nurses to have a 'buddy' or be buddies themselves is sound nursing practice. A buddy is usually a senior student who is able to offer additional support to a more junior student. The 'buddy system', which is a cooperative practice of pairing two people together, is often used to support learning in the clinical practice environment. Being a buddy while still a student prepares you to meet the requirement of the lifelong nursing commitment to support and teach others (NMC 2008).

All universities have a student support service that is able to offer support on a variety of problems a student may encounter, such as counselling needs, financial guidance, and study support. For example, the University of Nottingham has a financial support mechanism for students including a 'money doctor'. Students can arrange to see someone about short- or long-term money issues within the student services centre, or can post a question online to the money doctor.

Course information and professional behaviour

Horror! I didn't know anyone and what was being said scared the life out of me. I'd been out of education for a while and it shocked me how much was expected.

(Mental health nursing student)

I had mixed feelings. I thought it was full of information essential to starting the course and was very impressed; however I was daunted at the same time with the workload as they explained it.

(Adult branch nursing student)

I was nervous but really excited. There was a lot of paperwork and course info but this just built the excitement, I just couldn't wait to get underway.

(Adult branch nursing student)

The first day of your course is exciting but it can also be a drag. So much information is thrown at you it can be overwhelming, but just take your time to sit down at home and go through it again to make everything clearer.

(Adult branch nursing student)

Really, in the first week, it is all paperwork and photos for ID cards. Don't expect to do much studying the first week.

(Child branch nursing student)

Typically, the orientation process provides new learners with information about the course and a schedule of lectures or events they should attend. In sequence you will be introduced to information technology, library services, and academic procedures. Significantly, one of the unique requirements of healthcare courses is the need for professional conduct from day one.

We were expected to behave in a professional manner right from the start. We have to behave a certain way it appears.

(Adult branch nursing student)

The NMC (2009: 3) provides the following guidance on professional conduct to nursing and midwifery students:

It's important that, even as a student, you conduct yourself professionally at all times in order to justify the trust the public places in our professions. This can take some getting used to at first, but your tutors, mentors and the NMC are here to help you. Throughout your course you'll learn about the behaviour and conduct that the public expects from nurses and midwives.

The first few weeks of the course

This was no ordinary university course. There is an expectation of you from day one and this didn't become clear until the initial excitement had worn off and we really started attending lectures.

(Child branch nursing student)

It was daunting how much there was to learn but I wasn't as far behind my peers as I feared. I learned all about placements and what to expect; it was really great, and the preparation from the university made it really real.

(Adult branch nursing student)

Over the first few weeks we broke down into our smaller teaching groups, which allowed you to make closer bonds with other people on your course and made it easier for me to feel comfortable and ask the lecturer a question.

(Child branch nursing student)

Getting to grips with the quantity of lectures and work was quite daunting at times. I used to be absolutely shattered at the end of the day.

(Adult branch nursing student)

I found the first few weeks very tedious! For me this was the worse bit of the course.

(Adult branch nursing student)

New students experience what might be described as a 'torrent of information' in the first weeks of their course. Managing information overload is a difficult task and it requires the new student to become autonomous and independent in their approach to study. Strategies that may have been successful in your previous learning environments may not be as useful, and you will be encouraged quite early to develop essential study skills and use action planning/goal-setting.

Study skills and self-directed learning

I did some reading around self-directed learning and sought advice from websites. The course information, however, gave no guidance on self-directed study or on essay-writing technique.

(Child branch nursing student)

Self-directed learning is hard at times but still enjoyable.

(Mental health nursing student)

I'm fine with self-directed study as long as there is some type of explanation beforehand.

(Leaning disabilities nursing student)

I procrastinated a lot at the start of the course but I get down to it and use my time efficiently.

(Mental health nursing student)

I prefer working independently, so self-directed learning is fine for me.
(Child branch nursing student)

Adult learners are more self aware, can direct their own learning, and are motivated to learn by internal rather than external means (Merriam 2001) – in essence, they are said to be self-directed learners. You may be unfamiliar with the concept of self-directed learning but it is an inclusive process that should be offered to all adult learners at all levels of education (Quality Assurance Agency 2011).

Developing good study skills and habits will enable you to be:

- Successful
- Less stressed
- Manage your studies more effectively in relation to
  - Theoretical assessments
  - Placement achievement
- Ultimately achieve your goal of becoming a registered nurse.

(Williamson et al. 2008: 155)

ACTIVITY 2.2

Preparing to be a self-directed learner

- Read around the topic of self-directed learning to develop an understanding of what it means.
- Reflect on your previous learning experiences and think about what aspects of these involved self-directed learning.
- Consider how your previous experiences with self-directed learning have helped you.

Balancing nursing with home and social life

It has been difficult at times. I try to put nursing first, as it is what I will be doing with my life; however, I understand I need to take a step back and make time for myself to be able to keep focused on my nursing.
(Adult branch nursing student)

At times your free time is suddenly taken away and replaced with a shift pattern to work and studying to do at home and you feel you couldn't possibly fit anything else in. But you can by prioritizing and cutting yourself a little slack.

(Child branch nursing student)

When you are on placement your life can easily begin to revolve around work and nothing else, so organization is the key.

(Adult branch nursing student)

The course is very good – it is arranged in the same way as other academic courses, so I have been able to have an active social life as well as studying.

(Child branch nursing student)

Sometimes it can be difficult spending time with my son when I have assignments to do so I attempt to complete my university work when he is in school.

(Adult branch nursing student)

Nursing courses are different to most other programmes of study, as 50 per cent of the course is theoretical and set in the classroom while the other 50 per cent takes place within a clinical placement. In the university setting you will be required to attend lectures on weekdays, whereas in placement you will experience a variety of shift patterns. Nursing is fairly unique in that it attracts a broad age range of students rather than the traditional school leavers, so for some more mature students learning to balance nursing against a home and social life is essential. The importance of allowing time for oneself, friends, family, and others should not be underestimated. Activities such as having days out, listening to music, and going for a walk are all deemed to be of benefit. Nursing students who live in halls of residence will also experience some friction regarding integration with students on other courses, often due to the work patterns they are required to adopt. Some of the strategies used to integrate with other students are to join in student union activities and become a member of sports clubs.

Living in halls gives you an opportunity to meet new students, and hear about and be involved in activities, such as a night out.

(Child branch nursing student).

The biggest opportunity you have is in your first year when meeting new people. Joining sport teams, societies, and clubs allows you to mix with the whole student population. Your course does require you to do more work but it's just as important to socialize and take a break.

(Child branch nursing student)

When lectures finish at twelve we can to go to the pub for a few drinks. It may seem tame compared to other university students' activities, but it is enjoyable all the same.

(Mental health nursing student)

Managing finances

My bursary covers my rent, food, and mobile phone bill; other than this I rely on what I can earn through part-time work.
(Child branch nursing student)

It is a struggle but we seem to manage. I am also [registered with] a healthcare assistance agency, so I can do some shifts when needed.
(Adult branch nursing student)

Thankfully due to having a part-time job I am managing fine. It is important to think 'do I really need this?' when out shopping.
(Child branch nursing student)

I moved back in with my parents and do chores/help around the house in lieu of rent. It's not glamorous but it serves a purpose, as it means I can afford to study without having to work for the nurse bank as well, which would add more pressure to my studying.
(Adult branch nursing student)

Being careful with money is the key to survival. Due to having to work on assignments and placement it is not advisable to have a part-time job at the same time. I would not have survived without my free student overdraft; knowing you have that reserve should you need it can ease the strain.
(Child branch nursing student)

I am finding it a bit of a struggle . . . However I have to say the advantages of being on the course far outweigh the disadvantages of being short of money.
(Adult branch nursing student)

Managing one's finances is a very personal experience and while some students will manage just on their bursary payment, others require extra support from family members or via part-time work. Because nursing courses are intensive, you are not allowed to work more than 16 hours per month in addition to your studying. A significant number of students join healthcare agencies and work as a healthcare assistant for the duration of their course. Inevitably some students experience problems with debt and managing money. The university support services and student union provide excellent and confidential support for students and there are processes such as 'emergency loans' for those who require them.

The student finance services within the university are very helpful and give you all the help and advice you need.
(Adult branch nursing student)

Key points covered in this chapter

- How to select where you want to study and preparation for studying again
- How useful open days can be
- Guidance on applying for nursing through UCAS
- Tips for constructing your personal statement
- Help with applying for funding
- How varied settling into the course can be for students
- Exploring how you need to be motivated to make the most out of self-directed learning
- The importance of balancing nursing demands with your personal life

References

BTEC (2011) *The BTEC Level 2 Firsts in Health and Social Care.* Available at: http://www.edexcel.com/quals/firsts10/hsc/Pages/default.aspx

Department of Health (DH) (2011) *The NHS Bursary Scheme*, 12th edn. Available at: http://www.dh.gov.uk/prod_consum_dh/groups/dh_digitalassets/documents/digitalasset/dh_132640.pdf

Department for Education (DfE) (2011) *Directgov: Public Services All in One Place. Young People.* Available at: http://www.direct.gov.uk/en/YoungPeople/index.htm

learndirect (2011) *Qualifications.* Available at: http://www.learndirect.co.uk/qualifications/certificates/certificatesnumeracyliteracy/

Merriam, S.B. (2001) Andragogy and self-directed learning: pillars of adult learning theory, *New Directions for Adult and Continuing Education*, 89: 3–14.

NHS Business Services Authority (NHSBSA) (2011) *Bursary Scheme Information and FAQs.* Available at: http://www.nhsbsa.nhs.uk/Students/3255.aspx

NHS Careers (2011) *Entry Requirements for Nursing.* Available at: http://www.nhscareers.nhs.uk/details/Default.aspx?Id=1944

Nursing and Midwifery Council (NMC) (2004) *Standards of Proficiency for Pre-registration Nursing Education.* Available at: http://www.nmc-uk.org/Documents/Standards/nmcStandardsofProficiencyForPre_RegistrationNursingEducation.pdf

Nursing and Midwifery Council (NMC) (2008) *The Code: Standards of Conduct, Performance and Ethics for Nurses and Midwives.* London: NMC.

Nursing and Midwifery Council (NMC) (2009) *Guidance on Professional Conduct for Nursing and Midwifery Students*. Available at: http://www .nmc-uk.org/Documents/Guidance/NMC-Guidance-on-professional-conduct-for-nursing-and-midwifery-students.PDF

Nursing and Midwifery Council (NMC) (2010) *Standards for Pre-registration Nursing Education*. London: NMC. Available at: http://standards.nmc-uk.org/PublishedDocuments/Standards%20for%20pre-registration %20nursing%20education%2016082010.pdf

Quality Assurance Agency (QAA) (2011) *Assuring Standards and Improving Quality of UK Higher Education*. Available at: http://www.qaa.ac.uk

The Oxford Dictionary (2011) *Oxford Dictionary Online*. Available at: http://english.oxforddictionaries.com

Universities and Colleges Admissions Service (UCAS) (2011a) *Your Personal Statement*. Available at: http://www.ucas.com/students/applying/ howtoapply/personalstatement/

Universities and Colleges Admissions Service (UCAS) (2011b) *Applying to University or College*. Available at: http://www.ucas.com/students/

Williamson, G.R., Jenkinson, T. and Proctor-Childs, T. (2008) *Nursing in Contemporary Healthcare Practice*. Exeter: Learning Matters.

Further reading

Cotrell, S. (2008) *The Study Skills Handbook*, 3rd edn. Basingstoke: Palgrave Macmillan.

O'Brien, M. (2011) Overview of study and writing skills necessary to be an effective nursing student, in N. Davies, A.C. Clarke, M. O'Brien et al. *Learning Skills for Nursing Students*. Exeter: Learning Matters, pp. 21–39.

3 Getting the most out of your first placement

It's always going be scary doing something new for the first time, but try not to let nerves get the better of you. Try to stay positive, and don't let a bad first day put you off. I don't think I've enjoyed the first day of any of my placements, but you give yourself a chance to adjust to a new area. By the end of the placement I generally don't want to leave! Go with an open mind, expecting to get the most out of it that you can. You might be in an area which doesn't really interest you but that doesn't mean that there won't be anything for you to learn – sometimes there's just as much to learn about yourself and how you deal with situations as there is to learn about clinical skills. Most of all make the most of any opportunities that arise, and ask questions! (Adult branch nursing student)

Topics covered in this chapter:

- How you might feel in your first placement
- What you need to learn in your first placement
- The type of shift patterns you might experience
- How to make the most of the learning opportunities in your placement
- Understanding how your mentor can help you to learn
- Starting to apply your knowledge to the practice of nursing

Introduction

Starting your first placement can be a really stressful time, especially if you haven't worked in a healthcare setting previously. Even if you have previous experience, you will probably still be quite anxious about walking into somewhere new where you don't know anyone and are not quite sure what to do.

Before starting your first placement, your lecturers will have helped prepare you for your practice experience. You will also have had an opportunity to talk about what you might expect as well as some discussion time to talk through what might be causing you to be anxious.

It is always sensible to contact your placement area well before you are due to start so that you can find out what shifts you will be expected to work and who will be your mentor. If you are able to arrange a brief meeting it is useful to contact your mentor so that you know who you will be working alongside most of the time. This will give you an opportunity to start to establish a relationship with the person who will be looking after you as well as assessing your performance at the end of your placement.

Advice for students on their first placement

Try and experience as much as you can. Ask questions if you do not understand or want to know more. Don't worry if you get things wrong – you are a student and can't be expected to get everything right first time. Enjoy yourself. Yes, you are doing the course to learn and better yourself, but it also about the experience and making great friends.
(Learning disability nursing student)

Try and research into the area that you are going into before you start the placement. Discuss learning opportunities with placement staff and students. Don't worry about not being able to do anything, your mentor will know this is your first placement and will not expect you to run the ward. The staff are there to help and guide you.
(Adult branch nursing student)

Be willing to get stuck in and you will have a great time. I have come away with some like-minded life-long friends in that short period of time.
(Adult branch nursing student)

Don't be afraid to ask. The care assistants are a great source of information.
(Child branch nursing student)

Don't be scared. It is daunting but everyone is usually really friendly and willing to help. And have confidence.
(Adult branch nursing student)

Rely on your mentor – tell your mentor if you feel out of your depth.
(Child branch nursing student)

Be confident, but not cocky. Treat people – patients and staff alike – as you'd want to be treated. Don't be caught up in negativity; remember why you wanted to be a nurse in the first place. Get out there and grab hold of every opportunity you can to increase your learning. Value what seems like the 'boring stuff' like bed making, washing, observations, etc. It's great grounding and often provides a brilliant opportunity to talk to patients. Don't panic about the paperwork; give yourself two or three weeks and it'll start to make sense. Be the sort of colleague you'd like to work with!

(Adult branch nursing student)

Be inquisitive, the only daft question is the one you don't ask! Take a note pad everywhere to jot down questions, thoughts, and feelings. Keep a reflective learning journal and put in something learned every day.

(Mental health nursing student)

Key issues the students above identify include:

- make the most of any experience;
- don't be afraid to ask questions – staff expect this of you;
- talk to patients and learn from them;
- try to build up your confidence;
- talk to staff and be friendly;
- think about your experiences, reflect on them, and use your reflections as a part of your learning.

Getting to know the staff in your placement quickly is particularly important, since if you feel comfortable with people you are working with, you will feel more confident. This can be a crucial element in motivating you to learn and will also impact on how much you are able to learn (Chesser-Smyth 2005). If you are anxious and uncomfortable, you will focus your energies on those feelings, which will affect your ability to absorb new experiences and learn from them. If you are comfortable with people, you won't be afraid to ask questions that you think they might find silly. It is important to remember that everyone you work with will have experienced a first placement at some point, and most people will not have forgotten what that felt like.

How it feels to start your first placement

From day one, patients called 'Nurse!' and I wanted to run away when I realized they meant me. I was totally in awe and it took a long while to feel part of the team.

(Child branch nursing student)

I just had to throw myself in. For the first fortnight, I was like a deer caught in headlights, but I soon learnt I had to be confident – everything moves so fast, there's no time to be nervous!

(Adult branch nursing student)

I felt like an outsider and a bit of a fraud. I didn't feel I should be allowed to be doing the things I was doing, as I was no more qualified than someone off the street.

(Adult branch nursing student)

It made me feel proud.

(Adult branch nursing student)

Although you are excited about starting a new career, you are still nervous.

(Adult branch nursing student)

It felt good to be finally able to apply some of the academic learning to practice and to be able to help participate in the care of others.

(Mental health nursing student)

This is the first time I had ever done anything in the healthcare profession, so I was a bit bewildered but it didn't take long to settle in, as everyone on my first placement was so welcoming.

(Adult branch nursing student)

While you might feel a bit nervous, proud, and excited and at the same time a bit of a fraud, the only way to learn how to be a nurse is to do the job. If you have no previous experience, learning to do the tasks expected of you will help you to settle in and give you some confidence and this is often what a first placement is all about – helping you to feel like a nurse. Even having been a healthcare assistant doesn't guarantee an easy passage. Brennan and McSherry (2007) note that students can be in shock when confronted with the reality of nursing, and a previous healthcare assistant might suddenly realize what professional responsibilities are and escape from the pressures of being a student by once more adopting the role of a healthcare assistant. This might result in not accessing the learning opportunities you need as a student and can create problems in the long term. As a student, you need to learn how to become part of the profession, how to be a nurse, and how to use the learning opportunities available to you.

It is important that you develop a sense of belonging with the nursing team, because if you feel you don't fit in this can reduce your self-esteem and make you more stressed and anxious (Levett-Jones et al. 2007). It is worth spending some time getting to know people well before you put too much pressure on yourself to perform.

Becoming a professional

Through working alongside your mentor, you learn how to approach patients in a professional, yet caring manner. Through having your own experience, you then learn to communicate with children and their families.

(Child branch nursing student)

In my first placement, I learnt a lot by observing my mentor and the other nurses. I watched how they approached patients and also how they communicated with them. I tried to pick up on the phrases they used and the way they explained things to patients. Then I would try to do the same.

(Adult branch nursing student)

I come from a business background and used a lot of transferrable skills gained in business to working with patients and staff.

(Mental health nursing student)

One of the first things you need to learn is how to approach the staff and the patients in your placement. When you put on a uniform or enter into a practice setting as a student, you are viewed by the staff, the service users, and people's relatives and carers as a nurse and they expect you to act like a professional person. This means you need to adhere to the dress code for the area you are working in, be polite and courteous to others, as well as a punctual and reliable member of the nursing team. These things are really important in helping you to settle in and start to be accepted by those you are working alongside and those you are helping to deliver care to.

(Adult branch nursing student)

Adhering to the dress code and thinking about how you come across to people is important in learning to be a nurse. Members of the public expect nurses both to look and behave like professionals, and this will instil confidence in you as a nurse. The profession also expects you to present yourself in a particular way, and the Nursing and Midwifery Council (NMC 2009) provide guidance on the behaviour expected from a nurse when in university, in practice, and in their personal lives. As a nurse, you need to be polite and courteous, and aware of how you may be viewed by members of the public you come into contact with. Other key factors that students identify are observational skills, an ability to learn from your observations, role modelling yourself on nurses that you respect, and using your previous life skills experiences to help you relate to your patients/clients in a positive and productive way. Carefully observing how others act professionally will also help to develop and hone your observational skills when using them with patients/clients – a really important aspect of nursing.

Preparing for your first placement

My first placement was on the district team, so I got very lucky with the hours I was given. But I found it difficult doing a nine-to-five job five days a week.

(Learning disabilities nursing student)

I took things one day at a time, as childcare is a big issue for me; the actual shift patterns were fine – I loved it.

(Adult branch nursing student)

I coped well with shifts, and worked my family life, part-time work life, and social life around them.

(Mental health nursing student)

At first, the long days can be a shock to your system. However, working alongside your mentor can provide you with the best learning experiences on placement.

(Child branch nursing student)

I made sure I was organized in terms of preparing meals and was very boring and sensible about bedtimes and didn't go out much until I found my 'shift legs'!

(Adult branch nursing student)

As you can see, no single shift pattern suits everyone. Each person has different domestic demands and you need to have considered these responsibilities before you start your programme of study. It is really important to make the most of your time in placement with your mentor. You will be expected to follow your mentor's pattern of working as far as possible to make the most of your learning, putting him or her in a good position to assess you at the end of your practice experience.

Nursing is a really demanding course both physically and emotionally, so maintaining your health through sensible eating and getting enough rest are key. Expect to feel tired at first: feeling anxious and nervous will only add to your tiredness. This gets easier as you begin to feel settled and accepted by the team you are working with.

What you need to learn in your first placement

Basic skills – observations, fluid balance charting, infection control, personal care, communication – but also to gain an appreciation and experience of a patient's journey from admission to discharge.

(Adult branch nursing student)

How to deal with patients and how to deal with the paperwork side of nursing.

(Adult branch nursing student)

Communication skills, moving and handling.

(Adult branch nursing student)

Basic ward routines and consolidation of the things I had learnt in school, such as clinical skills and communication.

(Adult branch nursing student)

You are expected to learn how the ward works such as what time handover is, where equipment is stored and how it is used, whether there are any day jobs such as completing admission books.

(Child branch nursing student)

My mentor and I worked out in our initial interview where I would like to learn, and built a plan that enabled that to happen. The plan included things like care planning, observing medication being administered, and then developing an understanding of the drugs used and their potential side-effects, etc.

(Mental health nursing student)

My mentor expected me to know the basics of care but also to start trying to organize my workload and use evidence-based practice. I think sometimes my mentor expected too much of me but was understanding when I told her I was not comfortable with what she had asked.

(Adult branch nursing student)

The above students highlight key things that in their experience are necessary for you to learn in your first placement, apart from learning how to behave as a nurse:

- Essential care skills:
    - helping patients or supporting parents/carers with hygiene and toileting needs;
    - taking and recording observations on individuals;
    - moving and handling skills;

○ accurate record-keeping when filling in various charts and documents;
○ communicating appropriately with service users;
○ seeking and gaining consent before doing things to people;
○ communicating verbally and in writing to others.
- Safeguarding skills:
  ○ protecting people by taking appropriate infection control measures;
  ○ knowledge of medicines and their untoward effects;
  ○ how to deal with people, including observing them for signs of
physical or emotional harm.

The Nursing and Midwifery Council (NMC 2010) set out what you are
required to learn during your nursing programme and is quite clear that
in the first part of your programme you need to demonstrate professional
behaviour, be able to deliver essential care to service users, communicate
well, and be aware of how to safeguard individuals. It is also important to
discuss with your mentor at preliminary and intermediate interviews if
you feel he or she is expecting too much of you – it will be too late to do
this at the final interview. This shows how necessary a good relationship
with your mentor is so that you feel comfortable in communicating any
unease. It is vital to remember that as a student you may progress at a
different rate compared with your fellow students. There can be no set
prescription for the rate at which you achieve. What is important is to
demonstrate progress and to achieve what is required of you at set points
in your course.

Students highlight the importance of the preliminary interview in
terms of discussing what it is possible to achieve and using this as the
basis for planning how to do this during your practice experience. This is
especially important in facilitating a view of the patient's journey through
the healthcare system, as you may need to arrange insight visits to affili-
ated areas to gain an overall view. In addition, the whole of the healthcare
team can help you to get the most out of your placement.

Learning how to gain the most out of
your placement

*Ask! Staff are so busy, it's not that they were being unhelpful, but I knew
I had to take responsibility for my own learning. I saw various people
come and go from the ward and asked who they were and if relevant if*

I could spend time with them observing their role. My biggest tip would be to take an interest in what's going on and ask questions.

(Adult branch nursing student)

My mentor and associate mentor always tried to help me where they could and encouraged me.

(Mental health nursing student)

The healthcare support workers were absolutely invaluable.

(Adult branch nursing student)

During my first placement, the management students were very helpful and were able to offer advice that was current.

(Adult branch nursing student)

Because I was in quite a rural area for my community setting, I had a lot of time in the car with my mentor travelling from place to place. I used the opportunity to ask lots and lots of questions! I could use the time in the car to prepare myself for the next calls, too, so I would be thinking of what needed doing, what dressings I would need, etc. That travel time was quite valuable really.

(Adult branch nursing student)

My mentor took an active interest in helping me develop through actively helping me seek learning experiences and through his extensive network of contacts both on the unit and in the community among other NHS and third-sector organizations.

(Mental health nursing student)

Most of the ward team was very supportive; I could ask them anything, as many times as I wanted. I was supported by the link tutor from the School of Nursing who came to visit. I received great emotional understanding from the staff when dealing with dying patients, or during last offices.

(Adult branch nursing student)

Tutor support was the main support given. Since my placement was in a really small hospital, there were not any other real support links.

(Adult branch nursing student)

We have a student forum, link teacher rep, tutorials with personal tutors, associate mentor, mentors, befrienders.

(Adult branch nursing student)

Student forums, mentor, nursing staff, personal tutor and peers. Support was available via the link tutor and student union advice centre.

Additionally, students were encouraged to join the RCN and Unison, who offer support should it be needed.

(Child branch nursing student)

These students highlight the important role that different people play in helping to support you in making the most of your learning opportunities. The people they see as important in helping you are:

- your mentor/associate mentor;
- healthcare assistants/support workers;
- senior students;
- members of your peer group;
- student forums;
- link lecturers;
- personal tutors.

Students identified mentors as the key people in making their experience a fruitful one, but remember they are there to facilitate your learning not to spoon feed you information. Watch the experts at work and learn from how they do things and handle situations. When your mentor feels you are ready to undertake specific tasks, ask for feedback on your performance. Your mentor will then start to give you some responsibility by letting you do things by yourself, but you will still need to ask for help at times. Don't worry, this is normal and acknowledging your limitations is an important skill to learn in nursing.

A key thing to remember is to think about your experiences or the experiences you are about encounter so that you can identify what you know and what you might need to know about different situations/tasks/people/conditions. You can then tap into other people's knowledge, in particular that of your mentor, by asking questions that will fill in the gaps in your understanding. However, be careful to pick the right time – consider when you want to ask something if it is appropriate to do so. If the person you want to ask a question of is in the middle of dealing with a situation, patient or carer, they will probably not be able to give you an answer straight away. Use convenient/quiet times to get clarification of why things were done, or why they were done in a particular way for an individual. It is quite useful to keep a small notebook in your pocket to jot down things you need to ask or read up on so that you don't forget.

Care assistants/support workers are also an absolute wealth of information and knowledge and have often had years of experience in the setting you are in. It is well worth using their experience to help you make sense of your own experiences, and you may feel more comfortable approaching them in your early days in the practice setting.

Senior students are aware of what you need to learn and can be a tremendous help to you. In helping you to learn, it can also motivate them to learn and also gives them an opportunity to develop their teaching skills. Such an arrangement is called a 'buddy system' and is arranged formally in some universities (Aston and Molassiotis 2003). Your peers are also a key source of support and it is really useful to share and discuss experiences with them. You will be in different sorts of placements and talking through issues can help to expand your understanding of nursing and how you fit into the team. Some universities formalize this sort of peer support and arrange student forums and arrange times that students from the same cohorts can get together with a lecturer to facilitate the forum. This can be really helpful in reassuring you that other students feel the same as you do, and you can share different ways you have dealt with situations that have arisen. It also gives you the opportunity to ask questions and clarify things, such as what you really need to focus on in the type of placement you have been allocated to. Your link lecturers to the placement and your personal tutor can also help with this. Remember: they are there to help your development as a nurse and can be a great source of support and information.

Learning to apply theory to practice

I think the only person who can make the most of your learning opportunities is yourself. You need to have the enthusiasm to want to learn more and experience all that you can. I think the best way to learn while you are on placement is to try and get involved in as many things as possible and ask lots of questions!

(Adult branch nursing student)

I completed my portfolio, attended insight visits and talked with my mentor, but as I said before the care assistants were my main source of information.

(Adult branch nursing student)

The practice learning representatives based on the ward are able to inform you of development opportunities on the wards. However, during your initial interview with your mentor you are able to identify areas that you wish to develop.

(Adult branch nursing student)

My mentor had asked previous students to compile a list of useful short day placements that would complement my learning about caring in the community, and she supported me in arranging short placements in these areas.

(Child branch nursing student)

Having identified several areas of learning to be sought, my mentor was proactive in driving me to ensure I undertook and maximized my learning potential. This included gaining and sharing detailed feedback when I undertook familiarization visits to other departments or units.

(Adult branch nursing student)

Being on placement was great in that it helped to make sense of much of the theory I'd been taught to that point.

(Child branch nursing student)

It made things seem real. You can finally see how all the things you learned in the classroom actually apply to real life.

(Adult branch nursing student)

I questioned everything I did in placement and asked for support and always completed tasks with supervision.

(Adult branch nursing student)

This is something you learn to develop over time; speaking to other students can offer a different perspective on how to include theory and research into your nursing practice.

(Mental health nursing student)

I was encouraged to participate in the delivery of care and planning of care for patients using evidence and theory learnt in university. I was encouraged to ensure the principles learned were applied in every aspect of the patient engagement to engender a therapeutic relationship.

(Mental health nursing student)

Key points to remember

- Show enthusiasm for learning
- Take responsibility for your own learning
- Ask lots of questions to help you apply theory to practice experience
- Keep a portfolio of learning
- Read around subjects and issues
- Talk to your peers and other staff about what you are learning

Appearing keen and enthusiastic about a placement and what you want to learn will help your mentor and other staff that you work with to know what you need as an individual. It is really useful to discuss this before you start your practice experience, to talk through with your personal tutor or the link lecturer what might be appropriate. In addition, use the preliminary interview with your mentor to clarify what learning opportunities are available. You can then think about things that have been discussed and start to take responsibility for your own learning. The problem is that it is difficult to control the practice learning environment. Lots of different stimuli can make it difficult for you to pick up the essentials that you need to learn, but the only way you can learn about nursing is by doing and the more placements you have the more comfortable you will become with the work of nursing (Papp et al. 2003). Even if you make mistakes or you feel the experience was a negative one, you can learn from these about what to do or how to act in the future.

Working in clinical practice provides you with the opportunity to place your academic learning into the appropriate context, which is vital in helping you to make your academic learning and knowledge meaningful and useful to you as a nurse (Cope et al. 2000). Students identify how their theoretical learning started to make sense once they could apply this in practice. Unfortunately, service users often don't mimic textbook descriptions and asking lots of questions about what you have experienced, why things happened in the way they did, and reading about various topics will help you to make sense of your learning and the experiences you have.

Insight visits will help you to appreciate how the members of the healthcare team work together, and the sort of journey a patient has through the healthcare system. You need to identify what it is you want to get from the insight visit and feed back your experience and learning to your mentor so you can discuss how you can build on these experiences in the future.

You need to take responsibility for your learning and seek help and support from your mentor and other members of the team. Never take on more than you know you are capable of and get people to supervise you when doing anything you're not sure of. Keeping a portfolio of learning can help you to keep a track of what you learn and how you are progressing (see Chapter 7), and discussing experiences with other students can help to give you a different perspective on situations.

The key thing to remember in your first placement is don't panic! Learning to be a nurse is like putting together a massive jigsaw puzzle. The pieces don't seem to make sense at first but, as you work at it, they gradually start to take shape and form the picture that will guide you. As you gain nursing experience and work at your learning, things will begin to make sense and you will start to feel more confident, so don't expect this to happen overnight. This is the reason it takes such a long time to become a nurse.

Key points covered in this chapter

- What it feels like going on your first placement
- What you need to learn in your first placement
- Becoming part of the nursing profession
- Preparing for your first placement
- Making the most of the learning opportunities available
- Identifying who can help to you learn
- Starting to apply knowledge to nursing practice

References

Aston, L. and Molassiotis, A. (2003) Supervising and supporting student nurses in clinical placements: the peer support initiative, *Nurse Education Today*, 23(3): 202–10.

Brennan, G. and McSherry, R. (2007) Exploring the transition and professional socialisation from health care assistant to student nurse, *Nurse Education in Practice*, 7(4): 206–14.

Chesser-Smyth, P. (2005) The lived experience of general student nurses on their first clinical placement: a phenomenological study, *Nurse Education in Practice*, 5(6): 320–7.

Cope, P., Cuthbertson, P. and Stoddart, B. (2000) Situated learning in the practice placement, *Journal of Advanced Nursing*, 31(4): 850–6.

Levett-Jones, T., Lathlean, J., McMillan, M. and Higgins, I. (2007) Belongingness: a montage of nursing students' stories of their clinical placement experiences, *Contemporary Nurse*, 24(2): 162–74.

Nursing and Midwifery Council (NMC) (2009) *Guidance on Professional Conduct for Nursing and Midwifery Students*. Available at: http://www.nmc-uk.org/Documents/Guidance/NMC-Guidance-on-professional-conduct-for-nursing-and-midwifery-students.PDF

Nursing and Midwifery Council (NMC) (2010) *Standards for Pre-registration Nursing Education*. London: NMC. Available at: http://standards.nmc-uk.org/PublishedDocuments/Standards%20for%20pre-registration%20nursing%20education%2016082010.pdf

Papp, I., Markkannen, M. and von Bondsdorff, M. (2003) Clinical environment as a learning environment: student nurses' perceptions concerning clinical learning experiences, *Nurse Education Today*, 23(4): 262–8.

4 Support systems while on placement

> *If you don't ask, you won't know [what help and support is available]. Make sure you ask questions, ask anyone, mentors, colleagues, students, lecturers. Just make sure you know all you need to know!* (Adult branch nursing student)

Topics covered in this chapter:

- How to take responsibility for your own learning
- Developing ways of learning on placement
- How to recognize ways of learning in the classroom
- Learning with buddies, peers, and through learning forums
- How to access learning support from tutors and other healthcare professionals
- Continuing to work on your academic assessments while on placement

Introduction

Approximately 50 per cent of all pre-registration programmes in the United Kingdom are set in clinical practice; practice learning is an important part of the nursing curriculum. Supporting students while undertaking clinical experience is an important function for all those involved with the facilitation of pre-registration programmes: tutors, mentors, peers, and other healthcare professionals. Providing appropriate support will enable you to find your own way of developing independent learning strategies in the classroom and placement setting, thereby allowing you to take responsibility for your own continuing development.

How to take responsibility for your own learning

I am driven by a thirst for knowledge; I always what to know more. I think it helps to start with topics that really hold your interest and do some independent reading. I find this encourages me to branch off and look at other things.

(Mental health nursing student)

Without doubt, the best piece of advice I could give regarding being responsible for your own learning is to remember that the more you put in, the more you get out. I have found myself faced with a choice on many occasions of (a) doing some more research for that assignment or (b) going out with my mates and 'starting my research tomorrow' ... Of course, my life has changed because [for the moment] my priority is learning how to be a fantastic nurse. I still have a great social life, I still have lots of fun but I get all of my work done for my degree; a relatively small commitment of time now will pay back tenfold.

(Mental health nursing student)

I take responsibility for my own learning by keeping a reflective journal whereby I identify key aspects of my learning in the clinical placement and explore how I might approach the same or different experiences in future situations.

(Adult branch nursing student)

I make sure I am organized so that I am able to juggle all the different aspects of the course and placement. On placement in particular I arrange my own additional learning, for example visiting a different area, to meet the learning opportunities I am required to.

(Adult branch nursing student)

I spent a couple of weeks over the summer break looking at skills books about how I can get the most out of learning. This has helped me to be clearer on what my objectives are from doing this course. Now I've finished first year, I set my own learning objectives for a placement based on outstanding things from the last placement and my own specific interests.

(Adult branch nursing student)

In Chapter 2, you were introduced to the concept of the self-directed learner. Key concepts for successful self-directed learning included: organization, acceptance, enthusiasm, and motivation. All registered nurses, you will find, are actively engaged in self-directed learning to keep abreast of advances in patient-centred nursing care. Self-directed learning can take on multiple forms, including independent reading, journal keeping, reflection, and action planning. This is not an exhaustive list of methods of self-development, and perhaps you might prefer other ways of developing your learning, such as groupwork or self-instruction packages.

For successful self-directed learning, remember that it is easier to motivate yourself to learn about a particular issue if you find it interesting or if you have some form of assessment on it. Knowles (1975), a key author in self-directed learning, suggests that students should take the initiative in recognizing their own learning needs. Students can identify the resources they need, choose the appropriate strategy for learning, and evaluate their own progress. What you may find more difficult is prompting yourself to learn about an aspect you are less interested in or perhaps studying when you are tired. As a student nurse, you may be dealing with several different aspects of the course at the same time, such as working towards module assignments in addition to attending and learning in a clinical environment. Some of you will recognize opportunities and accept the responsibility for your own learning more quickly than others. Lecturers and mentors recognize that some people have a greater aptitude to self-directed learning styles than others, and will use differing approaches to support learning. What is perhaps most important is that as a student you carefully plan for your placement to get the most from the learning opportunities it has to offer.

How to plan for learning on placement

When preparing to go out and learn on placement, there are three broad principles you may wish to consider. These principles, taken from the Nursing and Midwifery Council's guidance for registered nurses on maintaining their personal professional profile (NMC 2008), promote a review of previous experiences to support the processes for developing new learning:

- Reviewing previous learning experience:
  - what has gone well?
  - what have you enjoyed?
  - what areas provide opportunities for development?
- Self-appraisal:
  - of overall performance;
  - of areas identified for development.

- Setting further goal and action plans:
  - identifying goals;
  - devising action plans;
  - reviewing outcomes, standards of proficiency, standards of competency achieved.

Preparing for placement, especially your first learning experience, may appear a daunting prospect but, as discussed in Chapter 3, there are people and resources available to help you. Some of the skills you require to nurse patients, such as taking and recording a temperature, will be introduced and practised in class, but setting goals and action planning before attending a clinical area are also important because what you need to achieve in practice is specific. Learning outcomes, or 'standards of competency', are laid down by the Nursing and Midwifery Council (NMC 2010). Most lecturers advise that you make an action plan that is SMART: specific, measurable, achievable, realistic, and time bound, to allow it to be useful and dependable. We would also recommend that when preparing for a placement learning experience, you take your action plan with you and speak to your personal tutor who has a role in supporting you with this activity.

My personal tutor has a significant role in offering me support with placement learning when required.

(Adult branch nursing student)

ACTIVITY 4.1

Writing an action plan

- Decide what you need to action plan: it could be for a placement experience or maybe some other activity such as a study plan.
- Look at available tools to help you identify what you need to include in your action plan, for example a SWOT (Strengths, Weaknesses, Opportunities, and Threats) analysis (Chapman 2011).
- Your learning organization may have information on analysis tools, such as SWOT, SNOB (Skills, Needs, Opportunities, and Barriers) or SNOT (Strengths, Needs, Opportunities, and Threats), but you may wish to look at other resources. For example, the website www.businessballs.com offers guidance and a free downloadable template.

- Read around SMART targets – make sure you understand what these measures are and how to use them.
- Show your plan to a tutor or colleague for feedback.

Developing ways of learning on placement

I learn best through doing. I like to be shown how to do something and offered guidance: to ask questions, to then take the opportunity to practise the skill myself, and subsequently receive feedback on my performance.

(Mental health nursing student)

I recently had a placement where I had two mentors with very different styles of support. This experience has enabled me to compare the styles, and I now realize I have a tendency to ask questions but that I actually learn best when the mentor questions me. Being questioned makes me think more about what I am doing and for the day when I will be qualified and have to make decisions.

(Adult branch nursing student)

I am a visual learner, so I like to observe. I monitor the qualities of members of staff in everything they do. I look at how they handle other members of the MDT [multidisciplinary team], I watch how they compose them selves with patients, how they deal with difficult situations, how they are on the telephone.

(Mental health nursing student)

Learning through observing, looking at available literature, and then hands-on experiential style of learning.

(Adult branch nursing student)

I learn best when I have a mentor who I can work closely with and who is a good role model for nursing care delivery. I also learn best in an organized and well-structured environment.

(Adult branch nursing student)

When on placement, I tend to read up on a particular diagnosis or nursing task when I get home and write notes about it and then, if I have any further queries, I ask my mentor for their opinion.

(Adult branch nursing student)

Learning in any setting is unique to the individual and the circumstances they find themselves in. Adult learners want to learn and they do their best when they feel free to choose their own direction (Rogers 1983).

It is important to remember that you are an individual and each learning opportunity is unique. In the practice setting, you will be allocated
one or more mentors. A mentor is usually a registered nurse who has
undertaken a further period of study to enable them to support and assess student nurses. The relationship between you and your mentor is
important; he or she will help you realize your learning potential. One of
the first roles of the mentor is to have an initial interview with you, in
which the two of you can discuss your previous learning experiences and
your action plan, in an attempt to assist you to build new knowledge and
skills. Mentors are experts in nursing care and are able to support you in
discovering and creating knowledge that is further embedded in clinical
practice. In following the example set by a registered nurse, you will be
using 'role modelling'. Following and learning from a registered nurse is
a very traditional but still acceptable way of practising the art of nursing, but should not be considered as the only way of learning. Student
nurses identify other key concepts in developing their learning, including
questioning skills – asking questions of others and being asked questions
yourself – and learning by doing.

Questioning

The importance of questioning as a strategy for student nurses is widely
acknowledged; asking pertinent questions is a means of motivation because interest is generated by both you and your mentor. A question and
answer session allows for instructions to be given and learning to be evaluated; it can, moreover, be used as a powerful method of encouraging you
as a student to practise using higher-order thinking skills. Questioning is
a cognitive activity (cognitive relates to acquiring knowledge by the use
of reasoning) and thus one of the primary means through which you can
develop your own meaning from a learning experience you witnessed or
participated in.

Experiential learning

Learning by doing is also a traditional way of developing skills and knowledge in practice, but rather than being an opportunistic way of achieving
practice outcome, there is a structured theory behind this method called
'experiential learning'. David Kolb is widely accredited with introducing
the term and defines it as the importance of experience in learning
(Rakoczy and Money 1995). Kolb considered that there was a sequence

or number of steps a student should follow to make sense of a learning experience:

1. A concrete experience (feeling)
2. A reflective observation (watching)
3. An abstract conceptualization (thinking)
4. An active experimentation (doing).

The benefit of this feeling, watching, thinking, and doing cycle is that you can start it at any point. The mental health student nurse quoted above commented that they learned by 'doing' or 'watching', thus highlighting how this process appears to work for them. This student nurse highlighted two separate starting points, and by progressing though Kolb's cycle produced the final knowledge from learning experience.

Having accepted that learning is unique to the individual and the situation, you would not be expected to choose a particular learning style; it is likely that your own practice learning experience will be one of a number of styles and approaches. However, if you need help with learning to learn, remember that your mentor is there to assist:

> My mentor identified the best learning style on placement for me, which I had already realized for myself. Each mentor is different, and I am starting to realize that I may have to learn different learning styles depending on which mentor I am allocated.
>
> (Adult branch nursing student)

Learning with buddies, peers, and through learning forums

> Buddying is a fantastic source of learning. There have been times when students in their first year – especially those who are experiencing their first placements – I have played a part in their learning, especially when they appeared to be struggling or needing advice. I was in the same situation in my first year and a third-year student provided massive support and information when it was needed.
>
> (Adult branch nursing student)

> On my first placement, I was with another student. This was a random allocation, and we got the most support from each other, especially with how to complete the paperwork. This was extremely useful.
>
> (Adult branch nursing student)

During one of my second-year placements I was on the same ward as a first year. It was her first ward and I remembered how nervous I had been on my first ward, so whenever I got the chance I would help her out, try and show or teach her something that she might not know. I think most of the students in my group want a more official buddy system, as getting support from someone who's been in your position recently is invaluable.

(Adult branch nursing student)

Buddy system – not officially, although one of my fellow students has been on placement at the same unit and when we overlap shifts we support each other, and via email at other times.

(Mental health nursing student)

I haven't been allocated a buddy on placement but I have made it my duty to befriend other students who are on placement to share advice and encouragement.

(Mental health nursing student)

Students identify that the buddy system:

- exists and supports learning in practice;
- is used either formally or informally;
- provides emotional support;
- can be used between students at the same point on the course;
- can be extended beyond nurse training.

Support between students at the same point on the course is often referred to as 'peer support'. It can also assist you to maximize your learning opportunities.

We bounce ideas off each other if we're unsure how to meet our outcomes. It's useful to get a different perspective.

(Adult branch nursing student)

I have developed relationships within my learning group and outside in the wider student nursing community with people I can turn to for advice and feedback, often through structured reflection. This is helpful to gain perspective on aspects of the course or placement, as often students are too close to the situation and unable to be objective.

(Mental health nursing student)

I have sought support from my peers especially when I am struggling to cope with certain situations. They provide a massive sense of support when it comes to certain aspects of healthcare, such as drug calculations and facing difficult times including the death of a patient.

(Adult branch nursing student)

There are some things from placement that you need to talk about, and your peers are sometimes the best people. Not only can they say whether it fits with their own experience, but they also understand the confidentiality issues.

(Adult branch nursing student)

Following our first placement, one of our tutorial sessions was dedicated to sharing an aspect of our experience of placement. This was of value as it helped the students to realize that although we all had differing experiences, there remains commonality from each of our experiences.

(Mental health nursing student)

One of my peers is a buddy, we always talk about problems while out on placement. We have also decided that we will continue this when we qualify.

(Mental health nursing student)

Learning with and supporting each other on placement quite rightly receives positive endorsement from students, mentors, and lecturers alike. Students are able to discus in tutorials how peer support helps them make sense of their own learning. Being helped by someone you consider has the same goals, fears, and anxieties is reassuring and helping others gives a great feeling of satisfaction. Helping others – whether another student or untrained professional – can also make you aware of what knowledge and skills you have actually gained. Sharing learning opportunities may be unstructured, by chance, but there may also be some formal systems of support with peers using a structured and shared strategy of reflection upon practice, something that is referred to as 'clinical supervision'. Sharing experiences, in a confidential way, is a widely recognized method of support and development for nurses. Many courses will offer you supervision or some kind of learning forum for sharing your experiences in clinical practice.

The Department of Health (1993:15) defines clinical supervision as: 'a formal process of professional support and learning which enables individual practitioners to develop knowledge and competence, assume responsibility for their own practice and enhance consumer protection and safety of care in complex clinical situations'.

We have forums on placement that are mandatory to attend and are displayed on the student board for practice placement. The information is updated by the practice facilitators in the hospital.

(Adult branch nursing student)

We had strong support on placement in a forum. We met at least three times for two hours each time and I found this useful to share positive and negative experiences.

(Adult branch nursing student)

I have experienced forums and received some valuable information from these sessions, including those provided by the practice facilitator and other students.

(Adult branch nursing student)

I haven't heard of a learning forum. Most of this form of support would come under informal discussions with other students on my course, which has been extremely useful.

(Adult branch nursing student)

I have had meetings with various mentors and tutors as well as class-room debates in relation to placements. This is very useful in that you can learn from your experience and grow as a nurse.

(Mental health nursing student)

I have shared my experiences with peers in feedback from practice sessions. This allowed me to see what others have done and made me think I would like to gain that experience next time.

(Child branch nursing student)

Learning forums are structured and confidential meetings between student nurses and a member of the teaching staff. The teaching staff member may set the meeting up and act as facilitator, but it is the students themselves who generate the topics to be discussed. Both positive as well as negative learning experiences are discussed, which can help students to feel valued as well as supported.

Seeking support from tutors and others

Sometimes talking over things you've seen on placement with your personal tutor can help you make sense of things and promote reflective thinking.

(Adult branch nursing student)

Sometimes it's useful to speak to a tutor; it all depends on the person that you get. I find some people are better at emotional support than others. I have found support from unexpected places, such as a tutor in the English department.

(Adult branch nursing student)

I believe that the personal tutor is a great source of support for all aspects of your university life. They help with personal problems, assignments, and placement issues. It is important that you feel they are approachable and trustworthy, so that you feel comfortable in telling them your problems.

(Mental health nursing student)

Although I can go to my tutor if I need to, I have a specific practice link person for each placement.

(Adult branch nursing student)

My academic tutor is somewhat removed from my clinical placements. My university operates a link tutor programme. This tutor is available to answer questions and provide advice while on placement and to advocate on the part of the student if necessary.

(Mental health nursing student)

Yes, I have sought advice, but I know that I can now ask doctors or any other part of the MDT [multidisciplinary team] for advice.

(Adult branch nursing student)

It is clear that you can obtain support on placement from a number of different people depending on what support you need. The list of people you might wish to consider includes:

- personal tutors;
- educational link tutors;
- practice support teachers;
- academic support;
- counselling services;
- members of allied healthcare professions, including doctors, physiotherapists, occupational therapists, and social workers.

Collectively, there is an extensive support system in place for your learning experience in a placement setting, from learning how to learn, to managing what you have learned, to how to share what you have learned with others.

Recognizing ways of learning in the classroom

I always learn better when tutors put things into context, so that we can better understand how concepts and ideas work out in practice. Although I dislike student led sessions and presentations, I do think that a certain amount of student input is valuable and encourages us to put in the work beforehand. That seems to be a good learning tool for me.

(Adult branch nursing student)

I learn best in groupwork – that way we can bounce ideas off each other and someone may introduce new information that some of us may not have known that is related to a specific topic.

(Adult branch nursing student)

I learn best in practical sessions, as this builds my confidence, and the lecturer observing the session can inform me if my practice is safe and accurate.

(Adult branch nursing student)

I learn best in small groups, with the same group of people. I'm a visual learner, so I find the anatomy display classes the best way to learn (where you have actual body parts to look at). I learn best in an interactive environment, for example, group discussions, which allow us to form our own judgements.

(Adult branch nursing student)

When I know the title of the lecture I am attending, I read around the subject before and after the session.

(Child branch nursing student)

[I learn best] through seeing things visually and in a logical order and practising in practical sessions.

(Child branch nursing student)

I learn well in smaller groups of 20 or so people; when in a large lecture theatre, it is hard to remain completely concentrated on the work in front of you. I like to work with other people and hear their opinions towards an issue. Although when it comes to assignments, I prefer to work alone at home.

(Mental health nursing student)

I am definitely a kinaesthetic learner. I learn best by doing. Everyone is different. Don't be put off by members of your cohort who get straight As in their exams and top marks in their assignments. I am super-focused and have never got an A in my life. It has become apparent that the best mode of learning for me is to (a) do the theory, (b) test the theory out by actually attempting it in a live situation, (c) refining what I understand to get my 'best practice'. To give you an example, I was a little bit worried about doing CPR [cardiopulmonary resuscitation] – I had managed to convince myself that I would never be able to remember what to do in that situation. However, If the course ever did have a 'show and tell *day', I would want to bring the lady in with me who collapsed while on the commode during my first placement who I managed to keep alive until the MET [medical emergency team] arrived. I didn't even have to think what to do, it all came naturally.*

(Mental health nursing student)

As mentioned previously, individual students have different ways of learning. Ways of learning are studied by lecturing staff and you may have completed a test in school or college to identify which learning style best fits you. One theory of how students learn is using one or more of a set of qualities or styles defined by Honey and Mumford (1983) as Activist, Reflector, Theorist, and Pragmatist:

- *Activists* – 'hands-on' learners, preferring to have a go and learn through trial and error.
- *Reflectors* – 'make clear to me' learners, preferring to have concepts explained before proceeding.
- *Theorists* – 'convince me' learners, requiring material to confirm that the information makes sense.
- *Pragmatists* – 'show me' learners, preferring a demonstration by someone who is seen as an expert.

Honey and Mumford's learning styles provide but only one theory of adult learning approaches. You may be more familiar with the terms visual, auditory, and kinesthetic learning:

- *Visual learners* – have a preference for seeing because they think in pictures; visual aids such as slides, diagrams, and handouts are helpful.
- *Auditory learners* – learn best learn through listening, as in lectures, seminars, and discussions.
- *Kinaesthetic learners* – are tactile and prefer to learn through experience and doing; projects and simulated practice are examples.

From experience it is likely that you will use more than one approach or style of learning, in essence selecting a method of learning that suits the material being studied. Lecturers delivering higher education programmes use a range of teaching methods, including lecturers, seminars, groupwork, e-learning, and practical sessions (a) to meet the curriculum aims and (b) to meet the varying types of learning students respond to. It is perhaps not surprising that student nurses state that they enjoy the more active ways of learning such as practical sessions and (small) groupwork because of the perceived hands-on nature of the course they have applied for. It is, however, important to remember that to provide good-quality care, you must be able to apply the appropriate theories to the skills you are practising.

Support with academic work

Our personal tutors are really good at supporting us academically. We get good supervision for written work, although there sometimes is a lack of consistency in the advice given by different tutors.

(Mental health nursing student)

The university actively advertises any support programmes such as academic skills and database searching to help build on our skills.

(Adult branch nursing student)

I've found all the avenues available at university for academic work as I've struggled with this at times. Use all the places that you are told about, and keep asking questions about where else you can get help if you still need some.

(Adult branch nursing student)

I am aware of the various study support that is available in the university as well as placement-specific courses that you can attend. It is easy to find help within the university, whether it is essay writing or the confidence building that you require.

(Mental health nursing student)

Yes, we have something called UPGRADE, which can help you with your structuring, presentation, etc., of work and gives tips on certain tasks such as referencing, doing presentations, and reflection. You can also go to your academic advisor for help and your seminar leader of that module.

(Mental health nursing student)

Yes, student support offers workshops such as referencing guides and writing essays. We have had lessons on using the library and searching journals. Also your personal tutor is always happy to help provide information.

(Child branch journal search solar)

The School of Nursing offers no assistance, and disabled student services are not able to offer course-specific assistance.

(Child branch nursing student)

Many students worry about getting help with their learning, but it is important to note that all universities offer a wide variety of support and you should not be afraid to request it. Academic modules or teaching units are supported by specific tutors or tutor teams and they will facilitate the direction of learning and support the assessment requirements. Personal or group tutorials (seminars) are a common form of academic support but not the only ones. Advances in technology mean more information can be made available online, for example podcasts and learning packages. A podcast is a digital (sound) or media (video) file and it is released through the web syndication used by the university in question. Podcasts and learning packages have the advantage of being easily accessible from a computer at a time to suit the student. If you undertake a quick web search, you will see that specific academic support is made available at universities. The following is an excerpt from the Student Services: Academic Support web pages of the University of Nottingham (2011):

> Welcome to the Academic Support web pages. We offer study support to all students, including those who are dyslexic or dyspraxic. Here you will find some information about the work we do and resources for your study.

Academic support is a free confidential service and can help with all academic skills, including planning for study and writing style issues. Academic support can also carry out assessments for either known or suspected learning difficulties, such as dyslexia. Following an assessment, they will make recommendations to the university regarding reasonable adjustments to support learning and, if necessary, arrange for learning resources (e.g. a designated laptop) to be made available to the student.

> *The academic writing service was superb. It was run by the English department; I got more support from them about how to structure an essay. This resource was invaluable for me and I've recommended this to lots of people.*
>
> (Adult branch nursing student)

Support with academic work while on placement

> *I accessed support in the form of guidance during essay writing. I wanted to check I was on the right lines. It was very helpful to have an objective, expert opinion.*
>
> (Adult branch nursing student)

> *My academic tutor is somewhat removed from my clinical placements. My university operates a link tutor programme. This tutor is available*

to answer questions and provide advice while on placement and to advocate on the part of the student if necessary.

(Mental health nursing student)

I have access to a few of the Trust's student learning courses that have run throughout my student career and they have been informative and a great opportunity to meet students from other universities.

(Mental health nursing student)

Found mostly left to my own devices.

(Adult branch nursing student)

The support made available to you while in the classroom setting is still available when you are on clinical placement. Some students either do not always recognize this fact or they focus more on the learning opportunities offered in the practice setting. Learning theoretically and in practice should not be separated but the fact that they often are remains a constant dilemma for all those involved in the teaching of nursing students. The most successful students are the ones who are able to bridge theory and practice by using the self-directed skills discussed earlier in this chapter.

Key points covered in this chapter

- The importance of self-directed learning
- The importance of making sure you develop your learning on placement
- The importance of applying your learning from the classroom on placement
- Making the most of your learning by learning from others such as buddies, peers, and through learning forums
- Making sure you seek help with your learning by using your tutors and other healthcare professionals
- The challenge of working on academic assessments while you are still learning on placement

References

Chapman, A. (2011) *SWOT Analysis*. Available at: http://www .businessballs.com/swotanalysisfreetemplate.htm

Department of Health (1993) *Vision for the Future*. Report of the Chief Nursing Officer. London: HMSO.

Honey, P. and Mumford, A. (1983) *Using Your Learning Styles*. Maidenhead: Peter Honey Publications.

Knowles, M.S. (1975) *Self-directed Learning: A Guide for Learners and Teachers*. Chicago, IL: Follet Publishing.

Nursing and Midwifery Council (NMC) (2008) *Personal Professional Profiles*. Available at: http://www.nmc-uk.org/Nurses-and-midwives/ Advice-by-topic/A/Advice/Personal-professional-profiles/

Nursing and Midwifery Council (NMC) (2010) *Standards for Pre-registration Nursing Education*. London: NMC. Available at: http://standards.nmc-uk.org/PublishedDocuments/Standards%20for%20pre-registration% 20nursing%20education%2016082010.pdf

Rakoczy, M. and Money, S. (1995) Learning styles of nursing students: a three year cohort longitudinal study, *Journal of Professional Nursing*, 11(3): 170–4.

Rogers, C.L. (1983) *Freedom to Learn for the 80's*. London: Merrill.

University of Nottingham (2011) *Student Services: Academic Support*. Available at: http://www.nottingham.ac.uk/studentservices/ supportforyourstudies/index.aspx

Further reading

Hutchfield, K. (2010) Getting ready to study, in *Information Skills for Nursing Students*. Exeter: Learning Matters, pp. 3–22.

Useful websites

www.businessballs.com/swotanalysisfreetemplate.htm
www.mindtools.com/pages/article/newTMC_05.htm

5 Issues when working on placement

> In the first couple of years, I would tend to deflect difficult questions to my mentor or other members of staff, and watch them as they delivered answers. I learnt a lot from that. Now that I'm in my third year, I feel a bit more confident in fielding questions. (Adult branch nursing student)

Topics covered in this chapter:

- Learning about professional boundaries between the nurse and patient/client
- Learning to deal with difficult questions from patients/clients and carers
- How to protect yourself in difficult situations
- How to cope if you have been asked to work outside your comfort zone
- How to develop your confidence in the practice setting
- Learning to be assertive on placement
- How to resolve difficult situations in the practice setting

Introduction

When training to be a nurse, half of your course will be spent in practice learning environments where you will learn to apply the theory of nursing to real-life situations. By working alongside registered nurses and other members of the team, you will learn to participate in the care that patients/clients require. Initially, you will be directly supervised but gradually that supervision will be reduced until you are able to plan and make decisions about patient care in collaboration with the patient/client and/or their carers. By working in clinical settings, you will be exposed to all sorts of situations and this can be quite daunting at first, for example learning to communicate effectively with patients/clients. You may be very good at communicating and developing interpersonal relationships in your personal life, but doing this in a professional capacity requires you to observe boundaries that you don't normally have to think about.

Learning about professional boundaries between yourself and patients/clients on placement

I learned from previous experience.

(Mental health nursing student)

I learned about boundaries from my mentors.

(Mental health nursing student)

Observing others and learning as I go through placements.

(Child branch nursing student)

I learned from trial and error really. Also from observing my mentors and fellow students and how they interacted with patients.

(Adult branch nursing student)

By observing other staff, by implementing learned communication models, by instinct and through experience.

(Adult branch nursing student)

I have read about and been lectured on developing therapeutic relationships with patients and how to engage/disengage. In placement I have read the patient notes and care plans for patients I come into contact with and have had the opportunity to speak to them.

(Mental health nursing student)

I used the NMC code, sessions at university, and by talking to other staff.

(Learning disability nursing student)

Trial and error, as I didn't feel I had support from the university.

(Adult branch nursing student)

I discussed what was appropriate with my mentor. She gave me examples, and quizzed me if I thought it was okay or not. I soon established that a professional relationship with a patient means you are there to support them, and although you may have a laugh and a joke with them, you are not to become too close.

(Adult branch nursing student)

It is important that you are made aware of people's quirks by other members of staff before you interact with clients. For example, some people may not like you to call them by a certain name or like to have their personal space. It is vital that you respect people's boundaries and that these can change as a client grows to trust you.

(Mental health nursing student)

I have read the NMC guidelines, which clearly state what the boundaries should be between myself and patients. I have spoken about this issue with mentors as well.

(Adult branch nursing student)

Key elements that the above students identify include:

- previous experience;
- observing and talking to one's mentors;
- observing other students;
- listening to and reading reports/handovers about patients;
- using theoretical learning applied to practice situations;
- gaining knowledge about the patient/client from available sources and how to approach them;
- professional guidance such as that provided by the NMC or the university.

Many students on nursing programmes have had some experience of healthcare prior to starting their course but for others their first experience of the nurse–patient relationship is on their first placement and this can be rather scary. Transferring learning from previous experiences is invaluable but all students work alongside other members of the healthcare team, with mentors and other students. You can learn so much by observing how they approach and interact with patients/clients. As you progress, it is important to reflect on your experiences to assess how well you or others have dealt with situations and how this might have been improved upon. Experience by itself is not learning. You need to examine what made interactions productive and incorporate this learning into your future practice.

Thinking about the experiences you have can also help you to make sense of theoretical knowledge you learn in university and can help you to utilize your knowledge in future practice. In addition, reading the patient care plans and paying close attention and asking questions at patient handovers will show you how others have approached situations, as well as what has worked well and what has not worked well in the past.

As a nurse, you also have to recognize and maintain appropriate boundaries in your relationships with patients/clients to protect any vulnerability on their part (Holder and Schenthal 2007). You must be professional at all times, since any boundary violations can harm the patient/client.

For example, you may really like a particular patient and, in building up a relationship with them, spend a lot of time with them because you feel at ease with them. They might offer you a box of chocolates because they appreciate your attention. But think about how this might be looked upon by others if you accept this gift, for example whether you cultivated the patient in order to gain something from them. You may even have unwittingly ignored other patients. The Nursing and Midwifery Council (NMC 2011) provide guidance on professional conduct regarding relationships with patients/clients. However, this does not mean you should not share some social contact with people you come into contact with on a professional basis. In fact, nurse–patient interactions often contain a social as well as professional component (Millard et al. 2006) but there are certain boundaries that cannot be crossed. You need to learn how to facilitate effective partnerships with your patients/clients without crossing the professional boundaries expected of you. This is why it is important for you to have good role models within the nursing team. If you are ever in doubt about professional boundaries, you need to talk to your mentor or personal tutor.

Maintaining professional boundaries is one aspect of learning to be a nurse. Another is acting professionally when patients or carers ask you difficult questions.

Learning to deal with difficult questions from patients/clients and their carers

In my first year I am typically not placed in a position where I need to do this independently. I have learned to be guarded in what I disclose to patients and how I handle questions pertaining to me personally.
(Mental health nursing student)

Always say you are unsure but will find out. Then make sure you do find out and inform them. If it is really tricky, get a registered practitioner to accompany you.
(Adult branch nursing student)

By taking the time to listen to the full question, you are able to structure a response; if you don't know or are unsure of the answer, say so! Parents will remember what you say, so be honest.
(Child branch nursing student)

Don't answer immediately and don't try to fudge it! Take advice from senior staff or your mentor and then go back to the patient with the answer; be honest and try to find out.
(Learning disability nursing student)

Honesty – if you do not know the answer, say that – they will appreciate your honesty. If it is a sensitive issue, such as a question about dying, I have always referred to a senior nurse.

(Adult branch nursing student)

To be honest, if I don't know then it's no use trying to guess and it can be a good learning opportunity.

(Adult branch nursing student)

This is something I have done an academic reflection on and it is something I aim to improve – my communication skills. This is a vital part of providing holistic care.

(Mental health nursing student)

Key issues these students identify include:

- protecting personal boundaries;
- being honest – if you are unsure, say so and don't pretend you know;
- finding out and providing feedback to the person yourself or observing your mentor doing this;
- using these situations as learning opportunities;
- reflecting on these situations and learning from them how you can improve your skills.

It is important to remember that on placement you are there to learn about how to do nursing. You are not expected to know everything. That is why you have a mentor allocated to you. He or she is there to guide you and to show you how to deal with difficult questions as well as how to develop other nursing skills. Patients trust nurses, and as soon as you start your training they will view you as a nurse. If you try to avoid questions or try to deal with situations in an ineffective way, you will lose that trust. Ask for help from someone more senior such as your mentor and observe how he or she handles the situation so you are better equipped next time. Make a note of anything you need to clarify and talk to your mentor later to make sure you learn from your experience. Also, ask for feedback about how you handled the situation and how you might be able to handle a similar situation better in the future. This will help to build your confidence and repertoire of skills, as nurses have to deal every day with difficult questions as well as diverse difficult situations.

Learning to protect yourself in difficult situations

By knowing my own limitations.

(Mental health nursing student)

By sticking to the strict guidelines of the ward, Student and NMC codes.
(Adult branch nursing student)

Having worked with people with challenging behaviour prior to coming into nursing, I have some insight as how best to protect myself and have received training to do so.
(Learning disability nursing student)

I learnt not to just agree and accept doing things which I was not totally comfortable with.
(Adult branch nursing student)

I always try to think before I speak. Remember that people can be in pain and under huge pressure. Try not to take things personally. Make sure I take time to reflect following emotionally upsetting times. Speak up if I feel things are getting too much.
(Adult branch nursing student)

Work as a team – reflect and learn from it.
(Mental health nursing student)

By not responding to violence or aggression from a patient or visitor, and escalating the situation. I read the situation to try to determine if I can deflect it, or calm it before getting security involved.
(Adult branch nursing student)

We have been allowed to take part in some self-defence training, which was fun but also very important to learn about. It is about being able to protect yourself from being in a vulnerable position and avoiding situations in which you might feel at risk.
(Mental health nursing student)

I always wore alarms and I always let other staff know where I was and what I was doing. In the community, I left my car registration number and mobile number and informed them when I was due to be back. I have never really had an issue. It's the same on the wards though, always let people know where you are going. Always think about what you are about to say and how it could impact on your patient.
(Adult branch nursing student)

Key issues include:

- gaining experience and learning from your experiences;
- patients often behave in different ways at times of stress or distress;
- get to know your limitations and recognize that if you feel un-comfortable about doing something, you must get help;

- learn to recognize signs that a problem is developing and try to defuse the situation;
- learn from the experiences and activities you have within the university;
- follow guidelines for safety put in place for you.

Nursing is always challenging, as people respond differently and can be unpredictable in how they progress physically, mentally, socially, and emotionally when ill or distressed. The way people respond is not usually directed at you personally, but how you respond or react as a person can influence the outcome of any situation. Gaining knowledge and skills from your time in university will help to equip you to some extent for the real world of nursing. However, consolidation of your learning in the university will come from the experience you gain from practising nursing. Observing what other members of the team do successfully will help you to develop a variety of strategies for you to use in your future practice.

You need to observe your patients carefully so that you can learn how to recognize that a challenging situation might be developing and you can take steps to prevent it. For example, if someone is becoming agitated or anxious due to their pain, asking your mentor to get an effective analgesic prescribed and administered early on may help to prevent the patient lashing out because they think no one cares and they are being ignored. It doesn't matter how busy you are, taking time to prevent/diffuse situations will help reduce the distress felt by everyone in the longer term.

You do need to recognize your limitations, however. If someone asks you to do something you are unsure of or you recognize a patient's agitation but don't know what to do about it, ask for help. Never try to deal with something you are unsure of. Such experiences are part of learning about nursing, and you are not expected to deal with everything you are confronted with. Remember, you might cause further harm by trying to get by rather than by asking for help and support.

Working outside your comfort zone

That's not always a bad thing, you need to push yourself outside that zone sometimes to feel like you have really achieved something.

(Child branch nursing student)

Working with patients who, because of their illness, are verbally abusive or aggressive is challenging, and I am learning to become more self-assured in my responses when this happens. I am confident in the mentor relationships I have that I am supported.

(Mental health nursing student)

Yes, within a low secure setting. I was frightened at first. The alarms took some getting used to.

(Mental health nursing student)

Yes, every day we have difficult situations on the ward. You learn to adapt quickly as a nurse and work through it as a team.

(Adult branch nursing student)

I had to look after a patient with dementia, and I found communication a bit of an issue. The patient could communicate verbally, and could chat about the weather for days on end. However, when it came to comprehending he was wet and needed his trousers changing, he couldn't get his head around it, and would lash out. I spent a lot of time with the patient in these situations, to reassure him we were there to help him, and were not simply trying to take his clothes off. With constant reassurance, getting the patient clean and dry was a lot easier.

(Adult branch nursing student)

I find trying a new skill is outside of my comfort zone for the first few times but I have never felt unsupported while doing it.

(Adult branch nursing student)

I believe that most of my placements have been outside my comfort zone but you soon adapt to deal with clients with challenging behaviours. It is a great feeling when you have exceeded your expectations and got through to a client who is particularly difficult.

(Learning disability nursing student)

It is clear from these students' experiences that you cannot develop competence as a nurse if you never accept challenges that are outside of your comfort zone. The key things that help you in these situations are to feel supported by members of the team, in particular your mentor. There is a great sense of achievement in successfully overcoming a challenging situation. The exciting thing about nursing is that no two situations are ever the same, and the more you expose yourself to new challenges and experiences, the more you will learn and the more confident you will become.

Developing confidence in your nursing practice

By getting positive comments about your abilities from staff, patients, and relatives.

(Adult branch nursing student)

My mentor's input really helps my confidence. When I feel like they trust me to carry things out, it makes me feel more confident in myself.

(Adult branch nursing student)

Feedback, positive attitude, praise, seeing results, contributing, and feeling valued.

(Learning disability nursing student)

Encouragement from tutor and mentor, being given the opportunity and responsibility to carry out tasks and interact with patients; just being prepared to get out there and get stuck in!

(Adult branch nursing student)

Being treated like part of the team – not just a student who is there because she has to be.

(Child branch nursing student)

By speaking to patients, relatives and staff, by confidently applying my knowledge to situations, and reflection on what I have done well and what I can improve on.

(Adult branch nursing student)

Working for a nursing agency to gain more experience ... mainly just continuing to practise skills. As a third year I still don't feel overly confident.

(Adult branch nursing student)

I believe that being able to talk to anyone is a massive bonus in this job, as you can instantly find something in common with a person, whether it's the football team they support or the place they grew up. Staff and peers can help you to grow in confidence by offering you guidance and encouragement.

(Mental health nursing student)

Being exposed to situations helps you to gain confidence. Putting yourself forward for things to gain exposure. Also repetition of tasks helps you to gain competency and confidence as you can then say, 'I can do that'!

(Adult branch nursing student)

Reassurance from my mentors and fellow students – especially from other students, because it is a great feeling to hear from someone on your level that they think you did a good job.

(Adult branch nursing student)

Key elements in building up your confidence include:

- positive feedback;
- trust;
- encouragement;
- being made to feel part of the team;
- communication skills;
- exposure to new experiences;
- constantly practising skills.

Positive feedback is of great value whether it comes from your mentor, other members of the team, patients or other students, as it helps you to feel valued and respected by the team. But positive feedback needs to be earned– first, you need to get involved and take note of any constructive criticism. So don't despair if you don't get lots of positive feedback straight away. With the right encouragement, guidance, and opportunity to repeat skills frequently you can become fluent in procedures and begin to develop true competence. Taking an interest in the people you are caring for will also help you to build good relationships and communicate effectively with them. So if you feel a little awkward with people to start with, chat to them about their lives and interests, as this will help to relax you. If you feel relaxed in an environment, you will settle more quickly and be able to learn more effectively.

In developing your confidence, you also need to learn to become assertive in your professional life to ensure you learn effectively.

Learning to be assertive about your learning needs

I find that asking questions is the best approach. If there's something happening that I want to see or experience, I ask if I can watch. The worst that can happen is that they'll say no! I find that most places are really open to students learning.

(Adult branch nursing student)

I am assertive when I need to be and have brought this into the placement environment. I do this through developing strong personal relationships with my mentor and the other staff I work alongside.

(Mental health nursing student)

Not every mentor is able to identify your weaknesses. If you don't feel like you are gaining from the placement, speak up or it is you that loses out.

(Child branch nursing student)

I'm not great at this, but having said that, I've never had a problem when I've asked to go on a visit or observe someone. I've just learned to be brave. So long as I'm sensitive to what's happening on the ward and show willing to work hard, it's okay to ask.

(Adult branch nursing student)

I always jump at the chance to assist in anything. I am also nosy and listen to all handovers and the nurses' conversations and hear what procedures are going to be done. Then just happen to be in the right place at the right time!

(Adult branch nursing student)

By completing evidence and telling my mentor 'I've done this, can you look over it for me please?' By asking my mentor if I can take two of my own patients and arranging insight visits.

(Adult branch nursing student)

I have learned to simply say, 'this is what I need to do, please can we arrange it at some point', and ask to observe things, or to carry out things when I know that something needs to be done!

(Adult branch nursing student)

As an adult learner I must take responsibility for my own learning, and identifying my learning needs with my mentor in placement helped to make others aware of what I wanted to achieve.

(Learning disability nursing student)

Being clear about what you want and need to learn is a good start to taking charge of your own learning. This is why the university encourages you to develop an action plan for your placement experience. In this way, you can set the scene for your experience at the first interview with your mentor. With his or her experience, your mentor can then help you to adjust your action plan to make it work in the time you have on that particular placement.

Developing good relationships and working at becoming part of the team is really important. If you feel valued and are comfortable within the team, it is easier for you to articulate your learning needs. It will also help you to say when you feel you are ready to take on more responsibility, such as being given one or two patients of your own to look after. However, if you feel your development is not progressing as it should or you feel you are missing out on learning experiences, don't leave it until after you have finished your placement to get help – it's too late then! If you feel you can't talk to your mentor, ask someone else in the team for help. Alternatively, if you don't feel able to speak up or have done so and nothing has come of it, then get some help from your link teacher or personal tutor. They will be able to support you in using strategies to make the most out of your placement and will do so tactfully.

Most students will have a trouble-free placement but sometimes difficulties can arise and you need to know how to cope with these.

Resolving difficulties in placement

I had a patient's relatives shout at me because they were unhappy with the person's diagnosis. I didn't react. I remained calm. I know it wasn't directed at me . . . I left them alone for a while . . . the relative apologized later and thanked me for understanding the situation.

(Adult branch nursing student)

The biggest difficulties I have had involved members of staff who don't always have the patience to deal with students. Thankfully, they are few and far between and there are always plenty of staff who are willing and able to teach.

(Adult branch nursing student)

I had some difficulty getting the right learning opportunities. I just got help and advice from the university.

(Learning disability nursing student)

Yes, with one mentor. It took quite a while to sort out and affected my confidence.

(Child branch nursing student)

I sought advice when faced with a difficult situation with my mentor. I wanted to check my behaviour was acceptable and was assured it was. I made a decision there were bound to be people I will find hard to get along with in my career, so I viewed it as part of my personal development. I didn't make a big thing of it, just stood my ground politely when necessary. By the end of placement the situation was much easier.

(Adult branch nursing student)

There are issues with some senior nurses who look down on you and seem to scrutinize everything you do.

(Mental health nursing student)

I had difficulty with a mentor who I didn't feel wanted me on her placement. I tried to seek help from the education rep in the area. However, this didn't seem to help and issues remained unresolved. In the end, I just kept my head down and learned how I didn't want to practise in the future.

(Adult branch nursing student)

If you are struggling to get on with them [your mentor] and this is affecting your placement, seek advice from your personal tutor or the education representative on the ward. I didn't speak to my tutor until after the placement, but had I said something beforehand I may have been able to change mentor.

(Mental health nursing student)

I have had problems with mentors, although they are usually just mis-understandings or they are stressed! I find that being able to talk to them about it is the first thing you need to do, although if it is something more delicate, the link tutors are there to support you.

(Adult branch nursing student)

Only a few of our respondents had difficulties on placement with patients and relatives. Keeping calm and not taking things personally, and allowing time for relatives to calm down helped the students to resolve such difficulties. As a nurse, you will come across people who are highly stressed and anxious, and it is sometimes easy for these people to blame those nearest to hand. Taking a step back and giving people time to calm down and assimilate information is often all you need to do.

Sadly for our respondents, most difficulties that arose involved mentors or members of the multidisciplinary team, which can affect one's confidence. Do seek help in sorting things out and check out with other staff members that you are not over-reacting, misinterpreting the situation or handling it inappropriately. If you don't feel a situation has been resolved satisfactorily, seek help from your contacts at the university and, if this doesn't work, talk to someone else in the university. Most universities have an escalation policy for any concerns students might have, so if you don't feel someone is helping you to sort a problem out, make use of this policy to get the help you require. Dealing effectively with problems with your mentor is essential in ensuring a good learning experience.

Key points covered in this chapter

- Learning about professional boundaries
- Learning to deal with difficult situations in practice
- Protecting yourself in difficult situations
- Learning to develop your nursing practice by working outside your comfort zone
- How to develop your confidence as a nurse
- The importance of being assertive
- Some pointers about how to resolve difficulties you experience in placements

References

Holder, K. and Schenthal, S. (2007) Nursing and professional boundaries, *Nursing Management*, 38(2): 24–9.

Millard, L., Hallett, C. and Luker, K. (2006) Nurse–patient interaction and decision-making in care: patient involvement in community nursing, *Issues and Innovation in Nursing Practice*, 55(2): 142–9.

Nursing and Midwifery Council (NMC) (2011) *Guidance on Professional Conduct for Nursing and Midwifery Students*. London: NMC.

6   Accountability issues

> *Acting according to standards and values, whether legal, professional, ethical or those I impose on myself. [It is about] being answerable and being able to justify my actions and omissions in a professional capacity.* (Adult branch nursing student)

Topics covered in this chapter:

- Understanding the meaning of accountability, responsibility, and confidentiality
- Recognizing how accountability relates to professionalism at work and in the social setting
- Information on using social network sites
- What patient confidentiality is and when to disclose information
- How to make entries in patient health records
- What to do if aspects of bad practice are encountered

Introduction

Nursing students are introduced early to the concepts of professionalism and are expected to uphold all the requirements of their professional body, the Nursing and Midwifery Council (NMC). There is a code of conduct for registered nurses and midwives (NMC 2008) and additional guidance (NMC 2011a) for nursing and midwifery students. This chapter will address the shared requirements of nurses in training and of registered nurses and some of the differences between them. Patient confidentiality and good conduct is expected at work and in the social setting. It is essential that all student nurses are able to understand and recognize how they can work to these standards and report appropriately when they have any concerns.

Defining accountability

Accountability is at the heart of nursing practice but is a fairly complicated concept to define. There are many forms of accountability and registered nurses are accountable for their actions and omissions (the things they decide not to do) in the following ways:

- professionally;
- ethically;
- lawfully;
- in relation to employer.

It is beyond the remit of this book to explore accountability in detail, so we have selected two definitions as a guide:

> Required or expectation to justify options; responsible. (*Oxford Dictionary* 2011)

> Professional accountability relates to the additional obligation of the professions not to abuse trust and to be able to justify their professional actions. Nurses and midwives are professionally accountable to the Nursing and Midwifery Council. (RCN 2011)

What does accountability mean to student nurses?

I am accountable for my actions, which means being responsible for what I do. During my placements, I am accountable to the university and my mentor, who is in turn accountable to the NMC.

(Adult branch nursing student)

Accountability is being responsible for every action, word, and move you make.

(Mental health nursing student)

To me it means being able to explain why I did something and take responsibility for the outcome as well.

(Adult branch nursing student)

To always be accountable for my actions and my decisions. Also being accountable for what I say. To be aware that for any discrepancies in my practice and bad practice I can be up before a court of law and the NMC.

(Mental health nursing student)

Acting according to standards and values – whether legal, professional, ethical or those I impose on myself; being answerable and able to justify my actions and omissions in a professional capacity. Doing the right thing.

(Adult branch nursing student)

As a student nurse, you are a member of one of the groups of people caring for patients who are unregistered and must be directly supervised, and thus you cannot be considered accountable in the manner defined above. You are, however, responsible for any tasks or duties delegated to you by the registered nurse. The NMC guidance for professional conduct for nursing and midwifery students (NMC 2011a) makes no reference to accountability, possibly because there is the expectation that student nurses work under the direct support and supervision of a qualified nurse. In contrast, registered nurses are accountable professionally, ethically, in law, and to their employer, and maintain this responsibility even when allocating tasks and duties to others (NMC 2008).

ACCOUNTABILITY

A nurse or midwife who delegates aspects of care to others remains accountable for the appropriateness of that delegation and for providing the appropriate level of supervision in order to ensure competence to carry out the delegated task.

The nurse or midwife remains accountable for the delivery of the care plan and for ensuring that the overall objectives for that patient are achieved.

(NMC 2011b)

Responsibility

It is sometimes difficult to distinguish responsibility from accountability; the two words are often used interchangeably, a point clearly emphasized in our respondents' comments. Responsibility may be expressed as the requirement to carry out an assigned task to its successful conclusion. What responsibility does not necessarily mean is taking the blame when something goes wrong. Working with responsibility as a student and with accountability and responsibility as a registered nurse is a distinguishing feature of the nursing profession. A professional who is accountable can be confident and assured of the standards of care they are delivering and supervising.

> *Being responsible, being answerable to a governing body, connected with concepts such as morality and ethics, having obligations to act and behave in line with a given code.*
>
> (Child branch nursing student)

Working as a professional

> *You are a 'student nurse first, and a university student second' was the message that has been instilled in us all the way through training so far. As a student nurse, you must not disgrace yourself. You must be a law-abiding, respectful human being. Outside of placement/nursing school we have a duty to uphold the reputation of the profession we are going into.*
>
> (Adult branch nursing student)

> *We've been taught very clearly that we are entering a profession and that we are expected to behave as such at all times.*
>
> (Adult branch nursing student)

> *We were referred to the NMC Code and given some information during a 'preparation for practice' lecture. To me, it was obvious stuff like not talking about patients, especially out of the placement area, being on time, being respectful to staff, adhering to the uniform code, and remembering at all times that we represent the School of Nursing.*
>
> (Adult branch nursing student)

> *We are constantly made aware of the issues that are in the Code of Conduct from the NMC. We have had professional accountability lectures and it is always brought up in assignments and tasks set in the classroom, as well as on placement.*
>
> (Mental health nursing student)

Professionalism and professional accountability will be introduced from day one and reinforced consistently in school and in placement. Good conduct is a prerequisite but you will find it becomes a natural part of your development as a student and then registered nurse. The NMC Code (2008) is an excellent resource for standards of good care and you should use this as a reference document; you can also visit the NMC website and telephone directly if you have specific questions. It is a topic that you should be respectful of but not afraid of, and you will find that the educational component of your course has the thread of professional accountability running throughout and you might also be given an assignment that focuses specifically on accountability in practice.

Conduct out of the workplace

Your professional attitude needs to follow you out of work. It means being more 'well-behaved' when out with friends having a drink, not that I wasn't well-behaved before, but I am definitely more aware of my actions now.

(Adult branch nursing student)

I think that you do need to be aware of the issues that come with being a nurse, especially if you are working within the area you live in. It is important not to let it become too much of a burden in your social life, while at the same time being aware of your responsibility.

(Mental health nursing student)

I would never do anything that would impact [negatively] on my profession. I would never behave in such a way that it may draw attention to me. I always behave, dress, and speak respectfully while out in public. I do at home as well, but I'm not in the public eye at home.

(Mental health nursing student)

My conduct is now no different to how I already did behave.

(Child branch nursing student)

We have a duty to help people outside of work if we come across situations where we can help.

(Adult branch nursing student)

Society has constraints on how we act as individuals and therefore your behaviour may be no different as a student nurse from how it was before. The values we have shape our individual approaches to life and our ethical standpoint. The important thing is that you are aware of the rules set by society and how they impact on you when representing the profession of nursing. Desirable qualities include:

- honesty;
- being non-judgemental;
- trustworthiness;
- reliability;
- respectfulness;
- helpfulness.

Social networks

There are 700 million users of the Facebook social network site worldwide (*Guardian*, 13 June 2011). The NMC (2011c) estimates 355,000 registered nurses and midwives have a Facebook account; the potential problem with this and any of the social networks is that of professional misconduct (NMC 2009).

> *I love Facebook but I am very aware about what to write and what not to write, as I worked in a school environment before I started my training.*
>
> (Adult branch nursing student)

> *The university told us to be careful with these sites and recommended literature to read. I am not a social network site user, as I think it is too dangerous to use these sites and be a successful nurse.*
>
> (Mental health nursing student)

> *I do use social networking sites, but I do not post about placements or anything related to the working environment and my profile is set to private so that you cannot see any information.*
>
> (Mental health nursing student)

> *I do occasionally use a social network site but I never put anything up about placements, lecturers, work colleagues or other students. We were also told never to do this.*
>
> (Adult branch nursing student)

> *Yes, I use Facebook. We were warned about not discussing anything to do with people we met in the course of our studies, whether patient, staff or student. We were advised to be careful about securing our profiles and posting potentially compromising photos.*
>
> (Adult branch nursing student)

> *I received lots of guidance from the university, and warnings of what has happened when things have been posted online. I rarely use networking sites.*
>
> (Adult branch nursing student)

> *The university has laid down very clear instructions on what we should/shouldn't be putting online. Basically, don't post anything to do with the course/university or placements. Even the most innocent of comments can be taken out of context so it's best not to say anything really.*
>
> (Adult branch nursing student)

The decision to join a social networking site is yours alone to make; some student unions actively encourage students to join the university or cohort sites to help with social integration. If you do use one or more social networks, it is important that you do take the time to read the written advice you receive on their use and ask the advice of others. One of the key reasons why social networking has to be taken seriously is because of the impact it can have. On average, each Facebook user, for example, has 130 friends and is connected to 80 community pages. There are reportedly 250 million photographs posted on the site every day. So posting something inappropriate has the potential to reach many people.

The 2008 NMC Code on standards of conduct, performance and ethics for nurses and midwives states that your conduct in real life and online will be judged in the same way and at the same high standard. Guidance (NMC 2011c) on what you should not write/post includes the following:

- confidential information;
- inappropriate comments about colleagues, patients, and others;
- comments that are intended to bully or intimidate others;
- sexual or inappropriate material;
- anything that is unlawful.

In addition, you should be careful how you use your social network site; consider marking it as private and never use it to form personal relationships with patients or service users.

Patient confidentiality

Confidentiality is the bedrock of a clinical relationship. That the information given by a patient to a nurse is given in confidence entails a duty of responsibility on the part of the nurse. Patients have the rights of privacy and self-disclosure and except in exceptional circumstances you should not disclose any personal information imparted to you.

> *You can maintain confidentiality, for example, by not speaking in front of other patients, by closing the office door, not leaving any patient documentation around, not disclosing information to others over the phone.*
>
> (Mental health nursing student)

> *I am always aware that you cannot use a client's name outside of the placement setting. It is important when writing essays that you adhere to this too. You have to relate confidentiality to yourself and think that*

you wouldn't want someone discussing your health with anyone you didn't want them to!

(Mental health nursing student)

Confidentiality is to not discuss patients outside the clinical setting and to be aware of whom I am discussing patients with in placement.

(Child branch nursing student)

Confidentiality requires that you keep records in a secure place; not discussing patient details with anyone apart from other healthcare professionals. I draw the curtains around the patient's bed if I am talking about something of a sensitive nature, keeping my voice low so other patients don't hear.

(Adult branch nursing student)

It may seem an obvious point to make but you should be aware of the links between confidentiality, consent, and record-keeping. Information you or another healthcare provider obtains from talking to a patient is to help in the planning of their care or treatment by a number of individuals. When you talk to patients, you should make them fully aware of how the information they provide you with is going to be used and who it may be shared with. Remember that as a student you will be working under the guidance of a mentor and he or she will be quite careful not to expose you to the most difficult of experiences. Patients also have the right to refuse permission for you to participate in their care, and if this is the case you should respect this and discuss with your mentor other learning opportunities for you.

Disclosure of information/breaching patient confidentiality

I had a situation recently in the emergency care department when I was talking to a teenager with suicidal tendencies. They opened up to me and told me a lot of background history as to why they felt so bad, but when the doctor arrived the patient wouldn't divulge this history to the doctor. After a discussion with the patient about what would get them the best treatment, they let me tell the doctor what had happened; of course, if the patient had refused then the situation would have been different. Thankfully, most people when they realize that it's in their best interest will let information be shared.

(Adult branch nursing student)

There are occasions when a patient may tell you something and stipulate that you must not share the information. There are some exceptions to the duty of confidentiality, as detailed below by an expert in aspects of ethics, law, and accountability, Brigit Dimond (2008):

- With the patient's consent
  - Legitimate to certain parties, for example spouse
- In the best interests of the patient
  - Patient may suffer if information not disclosed
- If a court order has been obtained
  - Child protection/subpoena
- By some statutory duties
  - Road traffic accident
  - Prevention of terrorism
  - Public health (control of diseases)
  - Abortion Act (Chief Medical Officer)
- In the public interest
  - For example, a lorry driver with epilepsy
- Under certain conditions to the police
  - May need court approval
- Under the Data Protection Act

This list of 'when to disclose' may seem daunting and we expect it will be difficult for you at the outset, as a student nurse, to recognize when you need to keep a confidence and when the information you have should be disclosed; it does become clearer with knowledge and experience. When being supervised, it is important that you discuss situations with your mentor or a qualified nurse. They will be much more experienced in this area and know when to disclose or how to seek further advice about a particular individual.

> *It depends what it was. If, for example, it was something that could affect their immediate health and put them in danger I would inform the relevant teams/healthcare professionals. On my mother and baby placement, I had a teenage girl who was heavily pregnant tell me she may try to kill herself. I obviously informed the nurse in charge. In the girl's and child's best interests, the information was passed to the mental health and safeguarding teams.*
>
> (Adult branch nursing student)

> *I would have to act in their best interests and if it was in their best interests to tell another healthcare professional, then I would have to do so; however, I would explain everything to the patient first and would only tell the relevant people if I thought it was necessary to have to do so.*
>
> (Mental health nursing student)

I would make them aware that if they were at risk, or someone else was, that we need to put things in place to protect them. It is important though that you try to maintain a trust between yourself and the client, even if the information has to be passed on.

(Mental health nursing student)

A valuable learning experience is to reflect on potential situations with your mentors and fellow students. There will be a time when it is you that has to decide whether it is right to disclose and to whom; previous experiences may assist you in your decision-making processes.

Learning to write in patient records

A health record is any record of information relating to someone's physical or mental health that has been made by (or on behalf of) a health professional. This could be anything from the notes made by a GP in your local surgery to results of an MRI scan or X-rays. Health records are extremely personal and sensitive. They can be held electronically or as paper files, and are kept by a range of different health professionals both in the NHS and the private sector.

(Department of Health Information Commissioner's Office 2011)

The NMC (2009: 3) determines that a record may be:

- handwritten clinical notes;
- E-mails;
- letters to and from other health professionals;
- laboratory reports;
- X-rays;
- printouts from monitoring equipment;
- incident reports and statements;
- photographs;
- videos;
- tape-recordings of telephone conversations;
- text messages.

Nursing records are the way we communicate the patient care we have planned, given, and evaluated; without written nursing records, patient care would be compromised. Information and skills for record-keeping (the term given to entering and storing records) will be introduced to you in lectures and reinforced in practice. As a student under the direct supervision of a registered nurse, you will be expected to record the patient care you have participated in in patients' health records. When making an entry, a registered nurse will provide a countersignature. The registered nurse is accountable for ensuring all record-keeping meets the required standards. It is important to note that records must be:

- factual;
- legible;
- written in ink;
- sequential;
- consistent, avoiding vague comments or phrases;
- free from jargon, abbreviations, and defamatory language;
- succinct;
- dated and timed;
- signed (name and designation of author added);
- stored appropriately.

There is a legal requirement to produce good patient records and to store them safely. It may be a good idea to spend some time reading up on this when thinking about record-keeping.

The need to record facts not opinion, the need for a second signature from a qualified nurse.

(Adult branch nursing student)

You need to make sure that your documentation is 'perfect'. This is vital in ensuring the correct care, medication, support, and information is given to whoever requires it. A mistake can mean you are putting the patient at risk.

(Mental health nursing student)

Not to be judgemental in your records, not to express any opinion, and always seek guidance from a qualified nurse to have your documentation countersigned.

(Mental health nursing student)

When writing records to be aware that we are still responsible for our actions, our mentor needs to countersign it, and it should be a factual record.

(Child branch nursing student)

On a couple of placements, I have been advised to write as if you had to stand up in court and justify what you have written. Don't put woolly descriptions, just state what you observe and the objective facts.

(Adult branch nursing student)

What you should do if you witness poor practice

I would like to think that I could go to my mentor and report it; thank goodness it hasn't happened yet.

(Adult branch nursing student)

Report what has occurred, possibly to personal tutors? I didn't observe any poor practice fortunately.

(Mental health nursing student)

Speak to the person concerned tactfully and/or refer to my mentor. If necessary, I would not hesitate to refer to the placement link person or School of Nursing staff.

(Adult branch nursing student)

I would inform my mentor and we would discuss what would be the best action to take. If it was something such as not using a slide sheet, then I would just bring this up [politely] with the person, but still inform my mentor.

(Mental health nursing student)

In the first instance, you should talk to your mentor or another member of staff or the ward sister might be the next option. This might not be possible though, so report to your personal tutor or the clinical area's link lecturer. Reporting is often difficult to do.

(Adult branch nursing student)

I have unfortunately observed some poor practice on placement and I felt I had to report it because my conscience knew it was the right thing to do. If you believe that someone is at risk or there is a problem within your placement or how it's run, you need to speak up. You do not have to worry about putting your job at risk; it is required of you to notice if anything is untoward.

(Mental health nursing student)

It is hoped that both as a student and registered nurse you do not experience poor standards of patient care, but it is essential that you are aware that problems may exist and know what you should do to uphold the reputation of your profession if you witness poor standards. The NMC (2008: 5) is quite clear about the responsibility of registered nurses with regards to poor standards of care:

You must act without delay if you believe that you, a colleague or anyone else may be putting someone at risk.

You must report your concerns in writing if problems in the environment of care are putting people at risk.

Both the employer and university will have guidance on what to do if there is a problem with the quality of care. If you witness poor care, it is essential that you give an account of what your concern is to the most appropriate person. In most cases, this would be your mentor or another registered nurse; the mentor/nurse will be able to investigate and provide a written report of your concern. In some instances, it may be necessary to contact university staff, such as your personal tutor. The processes for reporting concerns in practice will be made available to you by your educational provider and it is your responsibility to make yourself familiar with them. Reporting something or someone can be a difficult decision but any concern should be handled with sensitivity and you can expect to be supported throughout the process.

Conclusion

In this chapter, we have looked at what it means to be a professional and responsible for the way you conduct yourself at work and at home in the role of a student nurse. The NMC (2008) standards of conduct, performance, and ethics for nurses and midwives are there to guide you both as a student and registered nurse. We have addressed some of the key terms that underpin the profession, such as professionalism, accountability, responsibility, confidentiality, and record-keeping, and what actions you should take if you are witness to poor standards of care.

Key points covered in this chapter

- Understanding the meaning of accountability, responsibility, and confidentiality
- An exploration of the issues of how accountability relates to professionalism at work and in the social setting
- Being professional when using social network sites
- The importance of maintaining confidentiality and when it is possible to disclose information
- Key issues to take into account when making entries in patient health records
- The importance of reporting any poor practice observed

References

Department of Health Information Commissioner's Office (2011) *Health: What are Health Records?* Available at: http://www.ico.gov.uk/for_the_public/topic_specific_guides/health.aspx

Dimond, B. (2008) *Legal Aspects of Nursing*, 5th edn. Edinburgh: Pearson Education.

Guardian (2011) *Facebook Growth Slows for Second Month in a Row*, Monday 13 June. Available at: http://www.guardian.co.uk/technology/2011/jun/13/facebook-growth-slows-for-second-month

Nursing and Midwifery Council (NMC) (2008) *The Code: Standards of Conduct, Performance and Ethics for Nurses and Midwives*. London: NMC.

Nursing and Midwifery Council (NMC) (2009) *Record Keeping: Guidance for Nurses and Midwives*. London: NMC.

Nursing and Midwifery Council (NMC) (2011a) *Guidance on Professional Conduct for Nursing and Midwifery Students*. London: NMC.

Nursing and Midwifery Council (NMC) (2011b) *Advice by Topic: Accountability*. Available at: http://www.nmc-uk.org/Nurses-and-midwives/Advice-by-topic/A/Advice/Delegation/

Nursing and Midwifery Council (NMC) (2011c) *Advice by Topic: Social Network Sites*. Available at: http://www.nmc-uk.org/Nurses-and-midwives/Advice-by-topic/A/Advice/Social-networking-sites/

Oxford Dictionary (2011) *Accountable*. Available at: http://oxforddictionaries.com

Royal College of Nursing (RCN) (2011) *Accountability and Delegation*. Available at: http://www.rcn.org.uk/development/health_care_support_workers/accountability_and_delegation_film

7 Providing evidence in your portfolio to support your practice achievement

It is important that we are able to demonstrate an understanding of the theory behind what we do and how we apply this theory to practice. Creating a portfolio of the various forms of evidence ensures that we reflect back on what we have done throughout the course. (Adult branch nursing student)

Topics covered in this chapter:

- Exploring why you need a portfolio to support achievement of competencies
- Thinking about the sort of evidence you need to collect
- Explaining who will prepare and help you to develop a portfolio
- Finding out which reflective model students find most helpful
- Making sure you provide evidence for everything you have to achieve
- Tips for completing a portfolio of evidence

Introduction

Nursing is about delivering the most effective nursing to the individuals who come under your care. To do this, you need to demonstrate competence in the fields prescribed by the NMC (2010). What this means for you as a student is that you need to demonstrate that:

- you can do nursing skills;
- you deliver care in such a way that demonstrates respect for patients, their relatives, and other staff members;

- you know why you are delivering in a specific instance;
- your care and decision-making is based upon the best available evidence.

Why you need to collect evidence to support your practice achievement

To prove that you are a capable nurse. To show your understanding of what you know.

(Mental health nursing student)

It is a reasonably reliable method of displaying my competency in required outcomes. It shows development over time.

(Child branch nursing student)

Proof we have gained knowledge and considered our actions.

(Adult branch nursing student)

To show what you have done and what you have understood from that information.

(Adult branch nursing student)

Proof of achievement and to facilitate your own learning and development, and to show future mentors and lecturers the standard at which you are working.

(Learning disability nursing student)

You need to collect evidence to support achievements as practices in nursing change all the time. It demonstrates that you acknowledge this and aim to practise safely based on best available practice. Additionally, it aids students to examine their knowledge.

(Adult branch nursing student)

It is important to collect evidence because it can be beneficial in the long run when you are applying for jobs at the end of your training. It allows you to show your achievements and sell yourself to prospective employers.

(Mental health nursing student)

Key elements these students identify are:

- proof of achievement of safe practice;
- demonstration of your understanding of knowledge;
- development over time;
- aids critical thinking skills;
- aids decision-making;

- helps mentors to know the stage you are at with your learning;
- acknowledgement that nursing is changing all the time;
- helps potential employers to have an idea of how well you have developed as a nurse.

For you to enter the nursing register at the end of your programme, you have to achieve the competencies outlined by the NMC (2010) at the required level, and it is important that you demonstrate how you have achieved these. Although you will work alongside your mentor for much of your practice, he or she will not directly observe or be able to question you on everything you do. This is part of the reason you need to collect evidence that verifies what you have learned and undertaken. In this way, your mentor is able to take into account the whole of your experience in your placement and give you credit for the experience you have had with other members of the team.

As you progress your studies, you will move from being directly observed most of the time to being able to function by the end of your programme with minimal supervision. In addition, you will progress from learning about why you have to do certain things for patients through evaluating situations and the evidence available, before making nursing decisions about a person's nursing care. Reviewing how you develop over time will help you to identify actions you need to take so as to achieve your full potential.

Help in deciding what evidence to collect for your portfolio

There were specific lectures aimed around the subject and I was given an in-depth explanation of what would be expected to be included.
(Adult branch nursing student)

Lectures on portfolio construction.
(Adult branch nursing student)

We were given examples and opportunities to write a couple of pieces of reflective work to help us to prepare for placements.
(Adult branch nursing student)

Mentor on first placement.
(Child branch nursing student)

The student forums reaffirmed what was discussed in the portfolio sessions.
(Adult branch nursing student)

Reading associated info from the university and worked out for myself what would be of most use.
(Learning disability nursing student)

University tutors, students who are further into their training, ward staff.
(Mental health nursing student)

Personal tutor.
(Child branch nursing student)

A third-year student on placement gave me the majority of information.
(Adult branch nursing student)

The university will provide you with some guidance on how to complete a portfolio with examples of what you can use as evidence. However, it is not until you have experience in practice settings that you will identify the sorts of things you can use as evidence. Some universities use student forums in the first placement that are teacher facilitated. These forums allow time for peer support but also allow for questions you have about practice (e.g. how to start developing your portfolio) to be addressed. Your first placement can be a highly anxious experience, especially in relation to collecting portfolio evidence. As you can see from the above students' responses, mentors, other staff, other students, student forums, reviewing your lecture notes, and seeking advice from your personal tutor can all help to clarify which types of evidence will help to develop your portfolio.

If you are stressed about developing your portfolio, you will not be alone in this. McMullan (2008) undertook research into students' views on portfolios. She identified that the portfolio can cause a lot of stress if clear guidance is not provided. McMullan also identified that portfolios:

- provide evidence of how you work as part of the team;
- help make you aware of your strengths and weaknesses;
- make you think about what you are doing;
- encourage you to work at something you are not so good at;
- help to develop independent learning.

The sort of evidence you need to collect for your portfolio

Direct observation, written reflection.
(Child branch nursing student)

Reflection on practice, completed work products [anonymized], e.g. charts and notes, annotations of relevant research, articles or literature, notes from insight visits, witness statements from observed work by other members of the team, and documentation that shows your development.

(Adult branch nursing student)

Narratives, certificates, evidence, witness testimonies, essay and clinical skills passes in assessments.

(Learning disability nursing student)

I add work products, reflective writing, direct observations, reflective discussions, insight visits, and questions and answers.

(Adult branch nursing student)

I collect certificates from courses I have completed, feedback from mentors and tutors, good pieces of work that I have written, reflections, and anything that can support my study as a student.

(Mental health nursing student)

Certificates from training courses, learning diaries, reflections, significant events and what I have learnt from them. Evidence of documentation I have completed [anonymized] to compare my development through my training.

(Mental health nursing student)

Documentation from practice, information from reputable websites, policies, guidelines, and leaflets.

(Child branch nursing student)

Key pieces of evidence you can use in your portfolio are:

- observations of your nursing by your mentor and other staff;
- reflection on your practice;
- work products, i.e. written documentation you have to develop as part of caring for a person;
- publications, policies, and guidelines you have read as well as what you have learned from various websites you have accessed;
- notes about what you achieved on insight visits to other areas associated with your placement or when you have worked with various members of the healthcare team;
- commentaries from members of the team you have worked with;
- certificates of study sessions you have attended;
- university assessment records that show your nursing development and understanding;
- learning diaries.

What you need to think about when collecting evidence is what you have learned from your experience and reading, and how you might use your practice and learning to help you develop further. You need to document your learning and how you intend to develop further to provide you with some direction as to how to achieve your goals. A collection of articles or work products in your portfolio is not evidence of your learning, or even that you have read the articles. You need to demonstrate with each piece of evidence how you are starting to apply evidence to nursing-specific individuals or groups. The application of knowledge to your nursing practice is a key element in developing a portfolio. Reflection on your practice is also a key skill in developing and demonstrating your application of knowledge to nursing and your learning from the experiences you have had.

Models of reflection you can use to help you develop your nursing practice

I have used Gibbs' model of reflection, which is fairly simple to follow.
(Child branch nursing student)

Driscoll's (2007) model of reflective practice.
(Adult branch nursing student)

Gibbs, always. I know Gibbs now and can think about my reflection a lot before I write anything.
(Mental health nursing student)

I write a learning diary after every placement and any significant event.
(Learning disability nursing student)

As you can see from the above students' responses, Gibbs' (1988) and Driscoll's (2000) models are popular. There are, however, lots of reflective models, and your university might specify which model you need to use for your portfolio; others request that you use a model/framework that works for you. But it is important you use some sort of framework for reflecting on your practice. As you become familiar with your chosen framework, you can start to reflect by thinking about events/situations almost automatically, which helps you to start to question your experience and begin to work out strategies for developing your expertise. The key thing to remember in relation to reflection is what you have learned and how you have developed can continue to develop from your experience. Aston et al. (2010) provide guidance to help you explore this aspect further and how it relates to your practice experience.

Learning diaries are also a very useful way of helping help you to remember what you have experienced and any significant events. Take care, however, that they do not become a descriptive account. A descriptive account will detail what you have experienced but will not identify what you have learned from it, what you need to learn, how you can do something better or how you can transfer your learning from one setting to another.

Tips on collecting evidence to support your practice achievement

Think outside the box – there are loads of opportunities to meet placement competencies. See everything you do as a learning opportunity. Reflect each day on what you have learned and think how you can demonstrate this. Try to do some good-sized pieces of work, rather than dozens of little bits.

(Adult branch nursing student)

Ensure that you understand what is expected of you. The lecturers will explain if you have any uncertainties. Do some research to familiarize yourself with the practice competencies you are expected to achieve.

(Child branch nursing student)

Talk to your mentors, as they will provide guidance.

(Mental health nursing student)

Keep a diary of what you do each day on placement and try to allocate a placement competency to it. This acts as a reminder when you come to write a reflective piece or an insight visit record of learning.

(Adult branch nursing student)

Write everything down as soon as you do it in a little notebook and then reflect on that as soon as you can so your thoughts are fresh. It is amazing when you look at that little notebook at the end of a shift and see how much you have forgotten that you've done!

(Adult branch nursing student)

Read, research, record everything, you never know when it will be useful. Manage your time well, and always support your work with a rationale.

(Mental health nursing student)

Use work products, any patient paperwork filled in such as pre-op booklets, risk assessments. Photocopy and anonymize them, it proves you're doing it.

(Child branch nursing student)

Always back up the evidence with writing and make sure to keep everything confidential.

(Learning disabilities nursing student)

When collecting evidence try to use the most up-to-date research to support how you have achieved your practice competencies. The university website is a great way of accessing journals, books, and e-books.

(Mental health nursing student)

I would try and keep as much positive feedback as you can; photocopy everything and keep it safe.

(Adult branch nursing student)

From the beginning of your training keep a copy of everything, as you can edit out information as you go along.

(Learning disability nursing student)

Collect everything you do regards risk assessments. Of course, remove all patient details. Keep a reflective diary. Most of my reflection is in my head though. I think this is because reflection is about feelings too.

(Adult branch nursing student)

Collect information and then summarize what you have learned to show that you fully understand what the evidence you have looked at shows and how it can help you.

(Child branch nursing student)

A diary is more helpful than you realize.

(Learning disabilities nursing student)

Key tips for portfolio development include:

- develop your time management skills;
- ensure that all the evidence you keep maintains the patient's confidentiality;
- make your evidence as comprehensive as possible;
- if you are unsure about what to keep and record get help from mentors or academic staff;
- keep a diary/notebook that you can refer to later when you have the time to start collating evidence of your practice achievement;
- include how you felt about experiences;
- research evidence that relates to your experience to help you build up your knowledge base about nursing and the reasoning behind the actions employed in different situations;
- access all the resources provided by your university and practice areas;
- keep things such as thank you cards, as they can count as evidence too;

- don't leave gathering your portfolio evidence until near the end of your practice experience.

These tips are very useful. Although a lot of students say they think about their experiences in their head rather than writing them down, you will not be able to remember everything you have done and learnt when telling your mentor how you have achieved certain competencies and the knowledge you have developed to ensure you are delivering the best nursing care possible.

Start early on in your experience. If, for example, you have to complete an observation chart for a patient, you can make a replica copy to keep as evidence (no patient details included, of course). If you are then not sure how to develop this into evidence of your learning, ask your mentor, other students or a member of academic staff to guide you in how you can. Keeping a portfolio of learning is the same as learning any other skill – you need to practise the skill, and you may need some help in this at first. If you get advice and help early on in your course, you will quickly become familiar with the skill of portfolio development and will start to develop your own style in maintaining your portfolio. And using the resources that your placement and the university provide will save you a lot of time when examining why specific nursing care is necessary for a specific patient need/problem.

You may, however, be a little apprehensive about putting your feelings down on paper for others to see. Remember that parts of your portfolio do not need to be accessed by anyone else. However, if this is the case, you need to make sure that the 'public' part that can be accessed demonstrates enough evidence to assure your mentor that you have achieved all the competencies you need to achieve and to the required level.

If a patient or their relative gives you a personal card or thank you note, this is an acceptable way of providing evidence of your achievement. You will need to record the reason why you think you received it, and what you have learned from this. Of course, requesting such evidence would be unacceptable and unprofessional.

The evidence you collect in your portfolio needs to reflect your over-all learning and the competencies you have achieved during your pro-gramme (NMC 2010). You also need to map your evidence to the compe-tencies achieved.

Ensure the evidence in your portfolio covers all the competencies you need to achieve

Still learning that one.

(Learning disability nursing student)

Towards the end of a placement, I check which competencies I'm yet to achieve and then tend to ask advice on how I can meet them. This seems really contrived sometimes, but it's got to be done! Sometimes I reword a piece of writing, because I realize I've actually met more than I originally included in a reflection or piece of work.

(Adult branch nursing student)

Compare the evidence with the competencies.

(Child branch nursing student)

Use the explanatory document from the university, which gives examples of possible evidence that can be matched against each competency.

(Mental health nursing student)

I follow the competency booklet and keep it with me wherever I go so I can ask my mentor how I can achieve a competency if I am struggling to work it out. Mapping documents that are usually provided by your placement area are also useful guides.

(Mental health nursing student)

Choose the most important ones that you can cover well with sound evidence, as they will probably cover quite a few other outcomes if you support them with good rationales. Cross-reference everything, as this saves having a zillion pieces of work that all say basically the same thing.

(Adult branch nursing student)

Check with a mentor or other students.

(Adult branch nursing student)

By having a meeting with my mentor and discussing what I could do to show I have developed competence.

(Child branch nursing student)

I ensure that the evidence is specific to the areas that I am considering and is as up to date as possible to demonstrate understanding, knowledge, and best practice.

(Adult branch nursing student)

Familiarize yourself with the outcomes and do research on the placement. This will allow you to pre-empt the areas where you may struggle to achieve the competency or help you to get evidence for it so that you can put an action plan together and discuss any concerns you might have about achieving the competencies.

(Learning disability nursing student)

Link it with the domains of nursing and the nursing process. Look at your practice documentation to ensure they match a competency. Write supporting reflective diaries to clarify why you have included the information and what you have learnt from it.

(Adult branch nursing student)

By matching it on the grid the university give you.

(Adult branch nursing student)

When I start each year, I put up notes of what I need to achieve. This works well and then things don't pile up.

(Mental health nursing student)

I work through the competencies and make sure I have something as evidence for each one to show I have achieved it.

(Mental health nursing student)

Apart from showing yourself and others what you have learnt and how you are developing, your portfolio is a requirement for professional practice and provides evidence that you have achieved all the competencies required to progress on your programme. Your mentor will directly observe how you practise nursing but it is not always evident to him or her what you are learning and how you are working at developing your nursing knowledge and practice. This is why you need to develop your portfolio and the content needs to reflect your learning. It cannot be stressed too much how important the skill of portfolio development is and that it is a skill you need to learn and become expert at.

Key points to help you ensure you achieve all requirements are:

- reflect on the type of experience your placement will offer and plan what you think you can achieve before the placement starts;
- discuss with your mentor and other students how you can demonstrate achievement;
- use any mapping documents available, develop your own mapping tool or make notes as an *aide-mémoire*;
- use examples provided by the university or placement to help give you some ideas;
- think about what you have achieved and what is outstanding;
- develop action plans for what you need to develop and work on;
- make it clear what you have learned;
- quality is more important than quantity of material.

Making sure you have appropriate portfolio evidence to demonstrate your competency achievement means that you need to be organized in your learning. This is a good skill to acquire, as in clinical practice you will need to be organized in terms of delivering patient care. And, as a registered nurse, you will need to organize and manage others.

Your university will provide you with information about the practice placements you are allocated to and this can help you to start thinking about the learning opportunities you will have. You can begin to read about the sort of experiences and type of patients that you will help to care for. And you can then start to think about your personal action plan and goals you want to work towards before you start your placement.

Once on placement you will be able to discuss with your mentor what you think you will be able to achieve and which competencies you feel you might struggle to achieve on this particular placement. Doing this will allow your mentor to gain some idea of how organized you are and will also give him or her the opportunity to help guide you in achieving the competencies required.

As your placement progresses, recording evidence of which competencies you feel you have achieved will help also to highlight any deficiencies. You can then seek further guidance on addressing these deficiencies. Also, make explicit in your evidence of achievement how you think you are developing and learning, as this will help your mentor to provide feedback on your progress or lack thereof.

Lastly, remember that quality is better than quantity of evidence. A packed portfolio does not mean there is evidence of learning and development. If you are not explicit about linking learning from your experiences with your development, the portfolio is not going to assist your mentor in deciding whether you have achieved competence.

Key points covered in this chapter:

- Types of evidence that will provide evidence of your development and learning
- Support and help you can access to help develop your portfolio
- Reflective models that can help you to develop your practice
- Tips to help you develop your portfolio
- Making sure your portfolio evidence demonstrates how you have achieved all the required competencies.

References

Aston, L., Wakefield, J. and McGown, R. (2010) Using professional skills to support decision making: using reflection to learn from experience, in *The Student Nurse Guide to Decision Making*. Maidenhead: Open University Press.

Driscoll, J. (2000) *Practising Clinical Supervision: A Reflective Approach*. Edinburgh: Ballière Tindall in association with the RCN.

Gibbs, G. (1988) *Learning by Doing: A Guide to Teaching and Learning Methods*. Available at: The Geography Discipline http://www2.glos.ac.uk/gdn/gibbs/index.htm

McMullan, M. (2008) Using portfolios for clinical practice learning and assessment: the pre-registration nursing student's perspective, *Nurse Education Today*, 28(7): 873–9.

Nursing and Midwifery Council (NMC) (2010) *Standards for Pre-registration Nursing Education*. London: NMC. Available at: http://standards.nmc-uk.org/PublishedDocuments/Standards%20for%20pre-registration%20nursing%20education%2016082010.pdf

8 Transition: becoming a registered nurse

> *I think it will be a big shock when we finally qualify. Three years is not a long time and I'm positive that there will be things that we'll panic about, although I believe that I will have the confidence to practise in a way that will be beneficial to the NHS and hopefully become a valued member of a team.* (Year 2 mental health nursing student)

Topics covered in this chapter:

- How you can use your final semester/placement experience to prepare you for making the transition to becoming a registered nurse
- How to facilitate learning for others
- Deciding on an area to work in
- How to apply for a job
- How to prepare for an interview
- How to manage the change from student to registered nurse: preceptorship

Introduction

The final chapter of this book will focus on the end point of the course from the final undergraduate learning experience through to your first position as a registered nurse. Whether you choose to work for the NHS or in private healthcare, in the area you trained or further afield, the transition from student to registered nurse can be a challenge but one you can prepare for.

Making the most of your last semester and final placement

Up to the final semester or six months of your undergraduate nursing course, you will have focused all your energy on achieving your placement competence and academic awards. In the final six months (or possibly before this), your thoughts will turn to the fact that you have nearly achieved your ambition of becoming a registered nurse and that you will need to look for a job! Nursing courses are unique in that nurse lecturers and mentors spend considerable time in helping to prepare their students for employment. The final clinical experience or 'management placement' as it is often referred to must be no less than twelve weeks (NMC 2010) and has the potential, if approached correctly, to provide you with the knowledge and skills you will need as a new registrant.

I needed to develop my leadership and management skills. I wanted to work as a nurse would [but under supervision] and do everything that a nurse would.

(Adult branch nursing student)

Being able to function as a junior member of the team, with as much independence to carry out tasks and responsibilities as possible in the role of student.

(Adult branch nursing student)

Basically on the final placement to develop the skills that a nurse needs, so being able to delegate, time manage, communicate effectively, manage patients, act as a patient's advocate and in the patient's best interests, and work within a multidisciplinary team.

(Adult branch nursing student)

Becoming more comfortable in taking a leading role with patient care, for example assessments, medication (under supervision), and care planning.

(Mental health nursing student)

I think that it is important to get as much as you can out of your final placement and to work hard to achieve this. I would like to be able to understand the main workings of a ward environment and be able to hold my own in a multidisciplinary team meeting. I would also like to be able to work closely with other professionals as well as the clients to have an influence on each person's care.

(Mental health nursing student)

I think time management is a key issue in the final placement. Prioritizing your workload and being prepared for an unexpected event. Managing a case load of patients with decreasing supervision.
(Adult branch nursing student)

When registered, all nurses must be professionally accountable (see Chapter 6) and act with autonomy and confidence when participating in patient care at any level. Registered nurses must demonstrate the potential to demonstrate management and leadership skills at the point of preceptorship and beyond (NMC 2010). The Nursing and Midwifery Council define autonomy as follows: 'The freedom to make binding decisions, within the scope of practice, that are based on professional ethics, expertise and clinical knowledge' (NMC 2010: 144).

Management and leadership skills sound daunting and not something you might expect a senior student or a newly qualified nurse to possess, but by breaking down what these skills are we get a more reassuring and attainable list of qualities:

- To be able to work within a quality framework – that is, to adhere to standards and guidelines and deliver care based on best available evidence.
- To be able to prioritize patients', clients', or service users' needs.
- To make sound decisions based on critical thinking skills, which is the mental process of evaluating information, reflecting upon meaning, and examining the evidence before making a decision (Aston et al. 2009).
- To show leadership skills – or the process of moving a group or groups forward in some direction. To supervise others and contribute to overall service development.
- To work as an effective member of a team.
- To demonstrate excellent communication and interpersonal skills.
- To manage your time and that of others efficiently.
- To delegate when clear lines of accountability and responsibility have been identified and agreed upon.

In the final clinical experience, you will be working more independently with minimal supervision and will be expected to manage a small group of patients or clients. This will give you the opportunity to implement the key management and organizational skills listed above and as indicated in the students' comments. You can expect to be supported in developing these qualities by an experienced mentor and you should use your experience of leadership, organizational, and management skills to help you shape your personal statement in job applications.

Facilitating learning for others

In addition to leadership and management, another key skill of senior students is supporting others, in particular junior colleagues. Although buddying has been discussed in Chapter 4 as a valuable support system for student nurses, learning to support others at this point in your training serves a much more significant purpose. As a registered nurse, you will be expected to facilitate the learning of student nurses and others (e.g. care assistants) to become competent (NMC 2008).

> *Yes, I have been involved in teaching others and I now realize how much patience mentors have. It is not always easy to teach something that, to you, is so easy and like an everyday experience.*
>
> (Adult branch nursing student)

> *As a third-year student, you often get to delegate to and support other student nurses, especially first years – it helps you to learn how to deal professionally with other members of staff and let them manage their own workload.*
>
> (Adult branch nursing student)

> *Yes, I have been involved in teaching; it helped me to see that I do have the knowledge and communication skills necessary, so it gave me a boost in confidence in my abilities.*
>
> (Adult branch nursing student)

> *Teaching others makes you more aware of your own knowledge and also lets you see subjects in which you need to develop your knowledge.*
>
> (Mental health nursing student)

> *Whenever there has been a student working alongside me on the ward, I have always helped out with their clinical skills and academic work. I feel I am good at this and enjoy sharing my knowledge. I have also asked for support staff assistance when performing some parts of assessments. It was nice that the support staff asked me why I did this or said that and I was able to give a good rationale. It shows to me how much I have learned and it makes me feel proud that I am learning the skills and the knowledge of becoming a nurse.*
>
> (Mental health nursing student)

> *Teaching others has helped me to consolidate my own knowledge.*
>
> (Child branch nursing student)

For many nurses, one positive aspect of their role is the sharing of skills and knowledge. Student nurses in their senior years embrace teaching and supporting others. Teaching others and demonstrating practical skills allow student nurses to reflect on their own knowledge and achievements. The more they participate, the more confident they will become in their skills and abilities. It is important in your final placement that you not only embrace supporting others for the reasons given here, but also to assist you in your transition to becoming a registered nurse, associate mentor, and eventually mentor.

Looking for employment opportunities

Personally, I'd like a work area with plenty of variety and a fast pace. I'd also be attracted to somewhere where the staff work really well as a team.

(Adult branch nursing student)

An area I am interested in, with the benefits of a position in which I can further my career.

(Mental health nursing student)

Throughout my training I have had the opportunity to work in many areas and this has given me an insight into the areas that I most enjoy.

(Adult branch nursing student)

I would love to work within the acute wards for a couple of years to gain the experience needed to work further afield. However, in the long run I would love to go into art/music therapy to incorporate the degree I achieved before I began my nurse training.

(Adult branch nursing student)

Looking for employment would depend on travelling distance, the clientele, the staff, and the area. All these things really, as it has to be right for me [and my family].

(Mental health nursing student)

I want to work in A&E because I want to do the Tropical Nursing Diploma, which requires two years' experience in A&E. A&E also promotes prompt i.v. [intravenous medication] competence and paediatric resuscitation [the extra courses I want under my belt].

(Adult branch nursing student)

The area should have a supportive team, encouraging staff, show an interest in continuous development.

(Child branch nursing student)

The diversity of opportunities may be something that first attracted you to a career in nursing rather than altruism. Getting your first job is something you need to put some thought into. It has been said that nursing students probably spend more time planning a holiday than their first job! Think about this because you are in a good position to make an informed decision. The following are factors that are likely to influence your decision to make a job application:

- pay structure and promotion opportunities;
- staff and team dynamics;
- location;
- family and friends;
- travelling distance;
- reputation;
- previous experiences;
- field of interest;
- professional development opportunities.

ACTIVITY 8.1

- List the factors that will have an impact on where you would like to work
- Talk to people – your friends, your family, your tutor, and mentors
- If you have the opportunity, visit job fairs
- Look online such as www.nhscareers.nhs.uk
- Arrange visits to areas you may be interesting in applying to
- Try networking with healthcare professionals in the area you have an interest

---

Applying for a job

Be really honest with yourself about what you want from a job and what sort of area you want to work in. Do enough research before the interview stage so that you're more prepared. Talk to people who have been through it before just to get a better idea of what to expect.

(Adult branch nursing student)

Most universities will put on sessions or provide e-learning resources to help you with the process of applying for a position in nursing and it is well worth availing yourself of the help offered.

(Adult branch nursing student)

We've had a few sessions in university, but I tend to ask colleagues and friends who are nurses about their experiences just to see what it's really like. Our university is great in organizing mock interviews for us so that we can see what it is like.

(Adult branch nursing student)

My tutor has spoken about it to the group; other lecturers have mentioned it as well. I know there will be extra classes for CV writing and so on.

(Mental health nursing student)

Completion of a good application is vital to securing that interview and it continues to be a surprise that not all students give enough attention to this stage. Some advice would be to take a step-by-step approach to completing an application, and many of the student nurses who have assisted in this book have identified the same processes:

Make a portfolio, learn relevant information for the area of work that may come up in the interview, and possibly prepare a presentation.

(Adult branch nursing student)

A good written statement about yourself and your achievements to support why you would be an ideal candidate for the job.

(Adult branch nursing student)

I also believe that you need to be able to sell yourself to a prospective employer. You need to be able to say what you are good at and what you feel could be improved in your work ethic. It's also important to be able to say how you would adapt to the transformation into a registered nurse.

(Mental health nursing student)

I already have a job. It is in an area I was very interested in and had my supportive practice there. They knew me and knew what I was capable of, so that helped. But because I loved the area and was passionate about it, I feel this shone through. I also talked to other colleagues about what I could expect from the interview.

(Adult branch nursing student)

Complete a professional development portfolio, an up-to-date CV. I need to make sure I prepare for the interview and research and read around the area I am going to go into. I need to prepare myself for questions that I may be asked. I need to think about what to wear, travel expenses, and whether or not the job is right for me.

(Mental health nursing student)

*A strong, evidence-based, and well-documented portfolio. Good refer-
ences. Evidence of enthusiasm and devotion to an area of work.*

(Adult branch nursing student)

Application process

Before you apply

Start work on the portfolio or the profile that you intend to take to
the interview, to showcase your professional development over the pre-
registration course. Update your curriculum vitae; this may not be needed
for the application process but you can include it in your profile. Think
about who you will ask to provide you with a reference and discuss this
with them.

Identify your knowledge, skills and attributes, and your strengths and
limitations. Give some thought to any transferable skills you have developed during your course and in previous work experience or charitable
work. Write a general personal statement (you can adapt this when you
need to be more specific). The Royal College of Nursing's information for
students on the NHS Knowledge and Skills Framework (KSF) (RCN 2007)
may help you with this. The NHS KSF (Department of Health 2004) is used
by employers to structure job specifications, and by prospective employees
to identify the knowledge and skills required of them. Take care with your
statement; get it checked for structure, content, and typographical errors.
Remember, your application needs to be good to get you an interview.

Completing an application

Most application forms can now be accessed online, and the larger Trusts
operate a clearing system for many positions. Some organizations, such
as in the private sector and the armed forces, provide paper applications.
Whatever process adopted, before you start the application read everything sent to you; in particular, study the job specification they provide
and tailor your personal statement to match what they are asking for. If
you are sent a 'hints and tips guide', don't ignore it.

If you have done the preliminary work, this stage should not take too
long or be too difficult but it is always wise to check the closing date and
return your application in good time.

Submitting your application

Make a note of the date your application was sent and who it was sent
to in case of any queries. It is also well worth checking your sent box to
ensure an electronic application has indeed been sent, and sending postal

applications by some form of registered post (e.g. special delivery). Retain a copy of your application and the job specification, as you will need to remind yourself of what information you have provided when you attend an interview. Keep everything together – your profile, curriculum vitae, and application notes – in readiness for preparation for your interview.

Preparing for interview

I researched the area I applied for. I asked others what I could expect at interview.

(Adult branch nursing student)

Our university offered us mock interviews; they were nerve racking but an invaluable experience.

(Adult branch nursing student)

The university has provided maths assessments to highlight if extra support is needed. They also provided practice interview sessions.

(Adult branch nursing student)

Because of the stage at which I am studying, I haven't really thought much about the actual interview process, although I know that there are services provided in the university to help you learn techniques and tutors who are happy to provide you with references to support your interview.

(Mental health nursing student)

I haven't prepared for interviews just yet, as I have things that need to be handed in soon, but come January, I will start thinking about possible questions. A good place to recap will be NMC – although the NMC has become engraved in my brain.

(Mental health nursing student)

Key points from this section are to practise interview techniques, listen to advice from tutors, mentors, and peers who have undergone this process, explore the area you have applied for, even if you have had a placement there, and to identify questions you may be asked. In some ways, as a student nurse preparing for an interview, you have some distinct advantages. Throughout your training, you will have learned about how to present yourself, such as when talking to patients, and how to complete an assessment – essentially a form of interview. Mock interviews with others and in front of a mirror will give you an idea of how you perform to a set of questions but there are other things you can do to prepare.

A number of adult and child field NHS working environments set a pre-employment medication and calculation test. The medication assessment may include drug calculation questions, such as working out how much solution to draw up for an injection. It may also test knowledge of the processes of administration, for example what you are required to do if a patient refuses a medicine. Numeracy in nursing and medicine management is a recurring theme in all nursing courses and the NMC Standards (2010) and assessments in your training will prepare you for a test should you apply for an area where this is required.

There are some commonsense but practical tips in preparing for an interview that you should consider. If you are not familiar with a particular work environment, it is good practice to ask if you can visit and look around. Visiting allows you to:

- look around the clinical environment;
- meet some of the existing staff;
- allow existing staff to meet you;
- ask any questions you may have;
- find out where you are to be interviewed so that you can prepare in advance.

It is also a good idea to think about what you intend to wear; smart casual is the accepted practice. Try your outfit on before you go to interview to ensure it is appropriate when you are standing and sitting down; for example, short skirts ride up when you are in a sitting position while trousers may expose novelty socks! Avoid too many accessories such as fashion jewellery and scarves; when you are nervous you may be tempted to 'fiddle' with them. Don't be tempted to chew gum prior to the interview for a dry mouth, as you may forget to discard it.

What you might expect at interview

There are many places you can look for information on what to expect at an interview. The following list is based on the *Nursing Times* (2011) guide:

- Goals
  - For the employer to select the best candidate
  - For you to convince the employer you will be a competent and compatible member of the nursing team capable of making a positive contribution to the organization
- Starting the interview
  - Common to shake hands
  - Make eye contact
  - Panel will introduce themselves

- Settling the candidate
  - Panel may use an open question, for example 'tell us about yourself/the training you have undertaken'
- Questions about the job
  - Why did you apply for the job?
  - What can you offer this position?
  - What appeals to you most about this position?
  - What would you say are your strengths and weaknesses?
  - Scenarios to test information/understanding of position you have applied for/professional accountability
- Tips
  - Stay calm
  - Think about your answers
  - Do not lie or exaggerate
  - Do not make derogatory statements about areas you have worked in or people you have worked for
  - Be positive in your body language and smile
  - Give examples to reinforce your answers if you are able
  - Do not ask about pay and conditions at this time
  - Prepare a question to ask the panel
- Closing the interview
  - Thank the panel
  - Provide them with a phone number for them to contact you with the outcome of the interview
  - State you look forward to hearing from them

There is one final thing to say about applying for jobs and more importantly going for interviews – if you are not fortunate enough to get the position, the next best thing is to request feedback. Your tutors and mentors will have briefed you that interview panels use a point system to score candidates against essential and desirable criteria; whether you have lost out by a few points or more, go and see them to identify how you can improve your interview technique for next time.

Managing the change from student to registered nurse: preceptorship

Preceptorship programmes were introduced widely in the 1990s as a way for students to acclimatize to their role as a newly qualified nurse. Initially, this measure was a recommendation, but its role in supporting nurses to achieve early competencies in knowledge and skills has all but made it a requirement – at least for NHS environments. Preceptorship is the term given to the period of time the newly registered nurse is supported by an 'expert' nurse in the environment they are working in. For student nurses, it may not feel too dissimilar to working alongside a mentor with the exception that your preceptor is your guide and therefore not accountable for your actions and omissions as a registered individual.

> *I think it will be terrifying! But it's just like starting a new placement; it will take a while to get used to, but hopefully there will be enough support available to make the transition easier. I'm only around five months away from qualifying and I'm just starting to feel like a nurse, which hopefully will help for the first day when I put on the blue!*
>
> (Adult branch nursing student)

> *Hopefully there will be a good preceptorship programme on the ward I will work on. As a management level student you get a good idea of responsibilities and it hits home what it will be like as a staff nurse.*
>
> (Adult branch nursing student)

> *I think it will be a very exciting time but there will also be an element of feeling nervous and even anxious. However, I do also expect it to be like any new experience in which it will take a few days to settle into a new role.*
>
> (Mental health nursing student)

> *It will be scary but I hope by then I will be more confident in my nursing. I feel confident now but I am protected by my student status. When I become a registered nurse I will not stop reading and using evidence-based practice to provide care. I will feel quite lost, however the university has said that they are always there for their students. I am due to qualify in September and will start applying for jobs in the preceding March. During this time, I will prepare myself physical and mentally for the transition using the university as my first port of call.*
>
> (Mental health nursing student)

> *In my final placement in the third year I will have my own patients, which will help my transition to a registered nurse.*
>
> (Child branch nursing student)

Becoming a registered nurse is what student nurses work towards but it only starts to sink in during the last six months or so of their course. Key concerns include whether they will have a positive preceptorship experience and any anxiety they may experience. It is beyond our remit here to discuss how potential employers run their inductions and preceptorship programmes, but it may be something that you should address when researching employment opportunities. Anxiety, anticipation, and excitement are normal emotions. Much like when you started your nursing course, people will be there to help you through this transitional period; the difference this time is that you will have an excellent peer network facing the same challenges as you. Friendships you make in nurse training do tend to stand the test of time. So the advice is to embrace preceptorship and face the challenges it brings, as highlighted by one student:

It will be difficult and stressful – I will probably feel like I can't cope, but really I can and I will have had three years to prepare for this ... so much to learn and develop ... it will be hard but I will get there.

(Adult branch nursing student)

Key points covered in this chapter

- Using your final experiences as a student to prepare you for becoming a registered nurse
- Learning to facilitate others' learning
- Thinking about your first post as a registered nurse
- Tips on applying for jobs
- Preparing for your first interview
- The importance of preceptorship in helping you to make the transition from student to registered nurse

References

Aston, L., Wakefield, J. and McGown, R. (2009) *The Student Nurse Guide to Decision Making in Practice*. Maidenhead: Open University Press.

Department of Heath (2004) *The NHS Knowledge and Skills Framework*. London: Department of Heath.

Nursing and Midwifery Council (NMC) (2008) *The Code: Standards of Conduct, Performance and Ethics for Nurses and Midwives*. London: NMC.

Nursing and Midwifery Council (NMC) (2010) *Standards for Pre-registration Nursing Education*. London: NMC. Available at: http://standards.nmc-uk.org/PublishedDocuments/Standards%20for%20pre-registration%20nursing%20education%2016082010.pdf

Nursing Times (2011) *Interview Techniques*. Available at: http://www.nursingtimesjobs.com/article/2563729/interview-techniques/

Royal College of Nursing (RCN) (2007) *Information for Students: Outlining the NHS Knowledge and Skills Framework*. London: RCN.

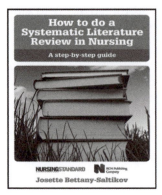

HOW TO DO A SYSTEMATIC LITERATURE REVIEW IN NURSING
A step-by-step guide

Josette Bettany-Saltikov

9780335242276 (Paperback)
January 2012

eBook also available

This is a step-by-step guide to doing a literature review in nursing that takes you through every step of the process from start to finish. From writing your review question to writing up your review, this practical book is the perfect workbook companion if you are doing your first literature review for study or clinical practice improvement.

The book features extracts from real literature reviews to help illustrate good practice as well as the pitfalls to avoid. Full of practical explanations this book will be invaluable at every stage. A must buy!

www.openup.co.uk

OPEN UNIVERSITY PRESS
McGraw - Hill Education